THE COMPLETE GUIDE TO
NAVY SEAL FITNESS

THIRD EDITION

Hatherleigh Press
5-22 46th Avenue
Long Island City, NY 11215
1-800-528-2550
www.hatherleighpress.com

The use of the words Navy SEALs does not imply nor infer any endorsement, either explicit or implicit, by the United States Navy or the Navy SEALs.

Before beginning any strenuous exercise program, consult your physician. The author and publisher of this book and workout disclaim any liability, personal or professional, resulting from the misapplication of any of the training procedures described in this publication.

Hatherleigh Press titles are available for bulk purchase, special promotions, and premiums. For more information, please contact the manager of our Special Sales Department at 1-800-528-2550.
Library of Congress Cataloging-in-Publication Data is available.

ISBN 978-1-57826-266-3

Cover design by Gary Szczecina
Interior Design by Fatema Tarzi
Photographed by Peter Field Peck with Canon® cameras
and lenses on Fuji® print and slide film

Printed in the United States of America
10 9 8 7 6 5 4 3

THE COMPLETE GUIDE TO
NAVY SEAL
FITNESS

THIRD EDITION
Updated for
Today's Warrior Elite

NOW INCLUDING WORKOUTS FOR ALL NAVY SPECIAL OPS RECRUITS, HIGH PERFORMANCE NUTRITION PLAN, AND THE PROVEN 12 WEEKS TO BUD/S PROGRAM

STEWART SMITH, CSCS, USN (SEAL)

PHOTOGRAPHY BY PETER FIELD PECK

HATHERLEIGH PRESS

NEW YORK

Here's what readers are saying about
The Complete Guide to Navy SEAL Fitness:

"I used this book to help me increase my endurance, and boy did it ever do that. My push-ups are stronger, as well as my sit-ups, and my 2-mile went from 12:27 to a 11:50 in a matter of just 6 weeks."

—a reader from Honolulu, HI

"A great fitness book, not just for SEALs! Probably the best exercise routine yet. LT. Smith's book takes you from warm up to burn out in 12 weeks. The diagrams are clear and concise, and the program itself is time-efficient and, most importantly, successful. For those needing extra help or motivation, Smith himself presides over a posting board at the publisher's website."

—a reader from Guildford, England

"This is the best SEAL training book available. I've reviewed other SEAL training books and LT. Smith's is the best. The 4-week workout builds strength and stamina, leading to the 12-week workout.

"Very well documented and true-to-life book that delivers an honest and pure approach to SEAL training...Bottom-line: GET THIS BOOK IF YOU WANT TO FEEL STRONGER, MORE DISCIPLINED & READY FOR ANYTHING IN LIFE."

—a reader from Coronado Naval Base, CA

"Greatest SEAL training book I've ever read . . . If you want to make it through the training then this is the only book you will need. It tells you about BUD/S, who to contact, plus every exercise you will need to do."

—a reader from Massachusetts

"Great book! Worth its weight in gold. I started LT. Smith's workout three weeks ago and am feeling great. I liked the variety of exercise that it offers. You can feel the burn the first day. It's great . . . Just a good old-fashioned workout, except one hundred times more intense! Great book if you want to be a SEAL."

—a reader from Madison, OH

"One of the better all-around workouts available...Smith does more with less in this book. It is an excellent way to get into awesome shape. He covers all the basics in the book, and takes them to new levels. Definitely a book for those who are looking into the SEAL teams."

—a reader from Mountain Home, IDC

"Excellent book for those serious about getting in shape...This is an excellent book for those not wanting to deal with weights or machines. I suggest that you start with half the reps that the book suggests and build up. I've been using it for three weeks and I'm already seeing definition in my abs and upper body. Sometimes simplicity works best and this book is a proof of that."

—a reader from Birmingham, AL

"The best workout I have ever done. Not for the weak. This book has helped me improve my level of fitness to a higher level. I am currently in the third week of the twelve-week routine. I am training for the NYPD. I am sure that I will be successful, as I will be prepared both mentally and physically. This book was a life-saver."

—a reader from New York, NY

"An excellent book for the advanced athlete...this is an EXCELLENT book for those looking for a challenging workout. I highly recommend this book for those going into the military or those interested in law enforcement."

—a reader from Mankato, MN

"I've had this book since the very first printing several years ago. Now, they include a DVD of all the exercises with it. Where else can you get one of the most excellent resources on fitness as well as a DVD? If you do the workouts included in the book, you will reach a level of fitness that you have never reached before. If you want to be in good shape, buy another book. If you want to be in GREAT shape, get this book."

—a reader from San Diego, CA

"I am in the last week of the 12 Weeks to BUD/S Workout and have just completed the max push/pull/sit-up day. I am so impressed. I have gone from only 7 pullups, 75 pushups, and 55 sit-ups at week one to 38 pullups, 125 pushups, and 80 sit-ups in week 12. I have lost about 15 pounds and I am in the best shape of my life. I love the fact that I can look around at the gym and I am confident that no one is working out as hard as I am. I am also trying to convert my friends to the workout, but I think they doubt themselves when I tell them about it. I even doubted myself when I looked at the workouts late in the program. This is a great book for anyone looking to lose weight, tone up, and gain a lot of strength."

—a reader from Virginia Beach, VA

"I was the type of kid in high school that did every sport I could; football, track, basketball, and heavy weight training. When I got this book I thought, 'This isn't going do anything for me.' Wow, was I wrong. I never felt this good in my life. Who would have thought pushups, situps, and pullups with swimming and running could get you in such good shape? This book is awesome. I advise anyone who has the work hard mentality to get this book."

—a reader from Memphis, TN

"I'm currently a sport science student and personal trainer, and I can safely say that The Complete Guide to Navy SEAL Fitness is an excellent book which encompasses all spheres of fitness in a stimulating manner."

—a reader from State College, PA

DEDICATION

The Complete Guide to Navy SEAL Fitness is dedicated to those men who have chosen a profession most men would not dare...

To those men who do every day what most men would not dream of doing...

To those men who understand what it means to "never leave your swim buddy"...

And to those who have given their lives in the service of their country.

HOOYAH to the US Navy Frogmen past and present!

ACKNOWLEDGEMENTS

How do I begin to say thank you to the many people who have helped me in the past, who have shown me the right path to follow in life? I could fill several pages with names of family members, friends, SEALs, and other Naval Officers and Enlisted to whom I am grateful.

First and foremost—my family has been absolutely supportive in all the endeavors I have chosen. Thank you Mom, Dad, and Liz for always believing in me when the chances were slim that I would succeed. You gave me the strength to TRY, which has led to my SUCCESS. My wife Denise, who has been with me since I was a Midshipman, has given me the will and the desire to strive for excellence every day. Denise and my new child have given me the energy and motivation to prepare for the future by working hard today.

My best friend from my hometown of Live Oak, FL—Keith Bonds has and always will be a friend, no matter how long I am away. Through his steadfast friendship and comic relief, I have learned to enjoy life by relaxing and watching the Suwannee River slowly roll past. My best friend in the TEAMS, LT. Alden Mills, and I have been together since we met on restriction our sophomore year at USNA. Through BUD/S, Advanced Training, SDV Team TWO Task Unit Alpha, and who knows what else, he has always been there for me no matter what.

The enlisted men of the SEAL Teams have made a huge impact on my life. Their dedication to duty and their loyalty to their shipmates has made an unforgettable mark on my work ethic and enjoyment of missions accomplished. Thanks for your energy! I wish I could list all of you, but I risk forgetting one of the many of you who has been my swim buddy, point man, or a good friend. You know who you are. The many senior officers, who lead by example, have made an impression that will last a lifetime. To my mentor CDR Tom Joyce—I have learned so much from your leadership and your example of what a Navy family should be.

I thank God for giving me the ability to accomplish what I have. With the strength God has given me, I can only hope to help others achieve their personal goals. That is why I wrote this book—to receive the rewarding feeling of helping another reach their goals.

—STEWART SMITH

CONTENTS

PREFACE

The Complete Guide to Navy SEAL Fitness has been a top-selling fitness book for over ten years. People with different backgrounds and goals have successfully used the workout to gain exceptional muscle stamina, cardio vascular endurance, and strength.

In this definitive third edition, the original 12 Weeks to BUD/S Workout has been left untouched. This plan continues to help Navy SEAL students graduate. In fact, recent graduates from the SEAL program were asked what they did prior to attending SEAL training and 85% of the graduating BUD/S class said they completed **The Complete Guide to Navy SEAL Fitness** and other Stew Smith fitness programs.

I developed the 12 Week to BUD/S Workout for midshipmen at the United States Naval Academy. In the two years, that the mids and I tested this workout, all thirty midshipmen who trained with the program made it through SEAL training. That is a 100% graduation rate in a school that has more than a 70% attrition rate.

After ten years, I can no longer boast a 100% graduation rate, as injuries, attitudes, and inability to handle cold water sometimes get the best of a fit BUD/S student. Everyone who has used **The Complete Guide to Navy SEAL Fitness** reported that they could meet the strict physical standards required. One thing is for sure: a SEAL career is not for everyone, and you will learn if you have the true desire to become a SEAL at BUD/S training.

Today more than ever, the Navy has realized that candidates attending SEAL training need to be in outstanding shape prior to attending BUD/S. There are now SEAL mentors in every recruiting district across the nation to help recruits prepare for BUD/S training. The Navy SEAL community is seeking to increase the numbers of the SEAL community by more than 20%. More people are pre-training for SEAL training than ever before. There are now cash bonuses available to those who graduate SEAL training.

If you are planning on going to SEAL training, do yourself a favor and complete the Twelve Weeks to BUDS Workout. This will not only prepare you for the BUD/S Physical Screening Test (PST) but for all the tough physical events of SEAL training.

The Complete Guide to Navy SEAL Fitness: Third Edition comes complete with instructional DVD to demonstrate many of the exercises, stretches, combat swimmer stroke, and teaches you how to run in sand. The new beginner plan in the book is a true beginner plan. A majority of today's applicants to a military profession will have to lose 20–30 pounds just to meet the basic height/weight/body fat standards. A smart nutrition plan has been added to assist you. These weight loss and fitness programs will be instrumental in helping you to avoid injury and insure success.

If you follow the plans in **The Complete Guide to Navy SEAL Fitness: Third Edition**, you will find yourself in the best shape of your life. This goes for men and women, young and old. Anyone can benefit from these workouts. If you cannot meet the repetitions and speed of the workouts, do what you can and you will still see phenomenal results. This workout will make you fail so you have to dig deep to continue. Therefore you will build mental toughness and be stronger the next time you do the workout. You will succeed by failing!

Hang in there and keep it up. I wish you luck as you begin to challenge yourself like you never have before.

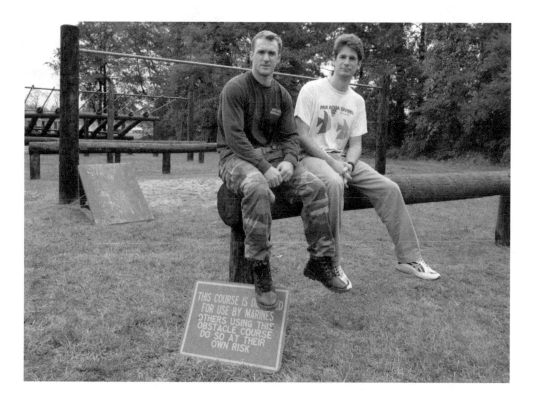

FOREWORD
TO THE REVISED EDITION

As with any product with a shelf life of ten years, time wins out and things must be updated. Several pages, a new nutrition chapter, and a new beginner workout have been added to **The Complete Guide to Navy SEAL Fitness: Third Edition**. Over the past ten years, this workout has helped thousands of people of every age become super fit—as well as helping a generation of SEAL candidates graduate BUD/S. The original 12 Week Workout is included untouched.

The Complete Guide to Navy SEAL Fitness is meant to be used two to three times in a year. That is only 24–36 weeks! In that time you will be amazed at the metamorphosis that occurs. After you have mastered this book, you may want to try **Maximum Fitness—The Complete Guide to Navy SEAL Cross-Training.**

FIVE PHASES OF FITNESS

If this is your first time picking up this book, here is the natural process of changing your life and becoming a new fit person.

1) Decision to get healthy / fit

Some will argue that it takes up to three to four weeks for something to become a habit. I say it takes three to four seconds! If you want to become fit, you will find every way possible to fit exercise into your schedule. Always remember, something is better than nothing. There will be days when you just do not have time to exercise an entire hour. Ten to fifteen minutes is better than doing nothing at all, so do some jumping jacks, pushups and stretches.

2) Doubt yourself

It is absolutely natural to have doubts about what you are undertaking. My advice is to start doubting yourself as quickly as possible and get over it. Realize that self-doubt is a natural part of the process of becoming fit and face it and move on. Even SEAL trainees doubt themselves, but those who conquer doubt become members of the elite Navy SEALs.

3) Conquer doubt

Now you have conquered doubt—you can do anything you set your mind to —is what you just told yourself. This is where the mind and body connect. Use the physical workouts to be a catalyst to energize other areas of your life: work, relationships, school. I am a firm believer that exercising your body gives you the stamina and endurance to exercise your mind, spirit and relationships to others around you.

4) Associate yourself with fit and healthy people

Now you are fit, you are comfortable in settings with young and fit people. Your example will inspire others to want to be like you. Your confidence in yourself will increase and open doors for you that you never imagined. People will be amazed by your work ethic at work and at play. Eating healthy is now a habit for you. In fact, eating fast food makes you feel slightly "ill."

5) Conquer a goal for yourself—whatever you like to do—run, swim, weight lift, or bike. Set a goal like running a marathon, finishing a triathlon, swimming a certain distance, lifting a certain amount of weight, or maxing out at higher reps of pullups, pushups, or sit-ups. Find a goal and get to it. This is a way to get into a mind set of competing—not just surviving.

To make it through BUD/S, you have to arrive on a day one ready to compete by winning races, PT tests, swims, and obstacle courses. Your goal should not be to merely survive each day. BUD/S is painful, but it is very painful if you are in survival mode.

INJURY DISCLAIMER

Before beginning any strenuous exercise program, consult your physician. The author and publisher of **The Complete Guide to Navy SEAL Fitness** disclaim any liability, personal or professional, resulting from the misapplication of any of the training procedures described in this publication. Take your health and fitness seriously!

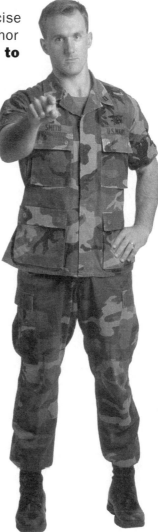

INTRODUCTION

THIS WORKOUT *WILL* PREPARE YOU FOR SEAL TRAINING *OR* ANYTHING ELSE!

Any well-conditioned person can do these workouts. There are over 70 different combinations of workouts included in this book, with pictures of stretches, exercises, running, and swimming. Over 150 pictures teach you every exercise as well as the proper techniques for running, swimming, and training with the world's fittest individuals—the US Navy SEALs!

You might ask, how does this workout prepare me for anything else? Believe it or not, if you can successfully complete this 12-week workout challenge, you will be physically prepared for ANY other military training. From Basic training—Army, Navy, Air Force, Marine Corps—to advanced military training like BUD/S, this workout will physically prepare you to do them all! Even if you have no desire to be in the military, but enjoy working out every day, **The Complete Guide to Navy SEAL Fitness** will definitely get you into top physical condition.

More importantly, the unbelievable amount of confidence you will gain in your abilities will change your life. Never before have you been able to do 750 pushups in one workout or complete the exhausting four-mile-run-one-mile-swim-three-mile-run in an hour and a half, but with this progressive step-by-step exercise program you will be conquering what you thought was impossible. You have no idea how this will affect your personal and professional life! You will gain confidence in your abilities that people will notice. Your boss, friends, and co-workers will see a lean, fit, self-assured person who has the attitude that anything can be accomplished. You will feel like you have never felt before in your life. You will have the energy to work all day, come home, play with the kids, or do whatever else needs to be done.

Let's face it. First impressions are lasting impressions. When you walk into a room full of people, the first thing they notice is your appearance—your height, weight, and physique. When you finish this workout, your physical appearance will command respect immediately; then, as you start mingling and talking to people, your words and actions will exude confidence. This is the biggest advantage you can have over your peers—confidence. Does this workout automatically give you confidence? NO! But it will help you build your confidence, just as it helps you build your strength and stamina.

PREPARING FOR SEAL TRAINING (BUD/S)

The primary goal of this workout program is to prepare and teach individuals about the challenges they will face at Basic Underwater Demolition/SEAL training (BUD/S). The secondary goal is to provide men and women with a progressively difficult 12-week workout that will challenge them every day. If you are a tri-athlete or a hardcore workout animal, you will enjoy this workout. THIS IS NOT A WORKOUT FOR BEGINNERS! You must be in shape long before you attempt this program. These workouts focus on running, swimming, and Physical Training (PT). PT, also known as calisthenics, is comprised of high-repetition, muscle- and stamina-building exercises that will make you leaner and more muscular than you have ever dreamed.

To achieve the primary goal of this workout, you have to be prepared to take the SEAL "Entrance Exam," also known as the SEAL Physical Screening Test, or PST. It consists of the following:

500 yard swim using the side or breaststroke	**(10 minute rest)**
Maximum number of Pushups in 2 minutes	**(2 minute rest)**
Maximum number of Situps in 2 minutes	**(2 minute rest)**
Maximum number of Pullups	**(10 minute rest)**
1.5 mile run in boots and pants	

This alone is a tough workout! Every fourth week during the 12-week workout, you will take the SEAL PST in order to check your progress. You may see that your scores do not change the third and fourth time you take the PST. This is because you are in the toughest weeks of the workout and are actually burned out (if you are doing all the exercises). But do not fear, because during weeks 10–12, a three-week tapering of intensity takes place and you will rebuild your strength and speed. After the twelfth week, start over at Week One and take the SEAL PST. After your three-week taper, you will see a huge increase in your numbers and a decrease in your times.

The three-week taper is in the workout in order to prevent over-training. If you are supplementing this workout with heavy weight-lifting workouts, longer swims, and runs during the "easy" weeks, you will NOT see the huge gains that a well-rested athlete will experience.

Below are the minimum times needed to pass the SEAL PST. As you can see, these scores are not that tough to achieve. However, a person who obtains just the minimum scores will not have a chance to get into BUD/S, due to the enormous competition of highly qualified applicants. The competitive scores are the above average scores that I have seen from men who get accepted into BUD/S. The best scores I have seen are from those incredible athletes you will compete with and work with when you are at BUD/S.

	Minimum Scores	Competitive Range	Best Scores I've Seen
Swim (min.)	12:30	7:00–8:30	5.45 sidestroke
Pushups	42	100–120	150
Situps	50	100–120	135
Pullups	8	20–30	42
1.5 Mile (min.)	11:30	8:30–10:00	7:45

Though there are no maximum scores for this "Entrance Exam," it is highly recommended that you give your best effort in all areas, in order to be competitive for this highly sought-after course of instruction.

Your number of pullups, pushups, and situps will increase after the 12-week workout. Your 1.5-mile-run time will decrease as you train to get your legs and lungs stronger than they have ever been. Your time for the 500-yard sidestroke or breaststroke swim will also decrease due to the large amount of swimming you will do. Detailed pictures and descriptions of the swimming strokes you will use at BUD/S will help you to perfect your technique.

BEGINNER WORKOUT PLAN

Many young men and women who want to attend Navy SEAL or Navy Special Operations training will begin their fitness quest by having to lose 20 to 40 pounds. It is more than difficult to run fast and perform pullups with this additional body weight. About the only thing you will excel in at BUDS with 20-40 pounds of extra weight is the float test—because you will be buoyant. To help with your quest, I've added a new beginner fitness plan and nutrition plan for weight loss.

This cycle will still have plenty of calisthenics, running, and swimming in the workout but will assist to create a stronger and fitter SEAL/Spec Ops Candidate. This new plan will help beginners to the world of fitness lose the necessary weight to make them competitive candidates AND make it safer for them to run and perform other body weight exercises.

ABOUT BUD/S

Basic Underwater Demolition/SEAL (BUD/S) training is one of the most physically demanding military programs in the world. BUD/S lasts for 26 weeks, with each week getting harder and harder. No one graduates from BUD/S without being challenged in some way. It is impossible to meet all the different demands of BUD/S without mentally pushing yourself to succeed. Graduating from BUD/S is possible (thousands have been successful), but ask any SEAL and they will tell you that something personally challenged them to dig deep within and push themselves to succeed. This is why BUD/S is called the "toughest military training in the world."

BUD/S is divided into three phases. Descriptions of each phase are below.

FIRST PHASE (BASIC CONDITIONING)

First Phase lasts for nine weeks. The first four weeks test you in the areas of soft-sand running in boots, swimming with fins in the ocean, and doing more pullups, pushups, and flutter kicks than you have ever imagined doing. On the average, a member of your class will quit each day during the first four weeks. The fifth week is known as "Hell Week." During this week, BUD/S students endure 120 hours of continuous training, with minimal sleep (a total of 3–4 hours—for the entire week). Also known as "Motivational Week," this week is designed to be the ultimate test of the student's physical and mental desire to become a SEAL. Typically, fifty percent of your class will quit or be medically discharged by the time Hell Week is over.

WHY DO HELL WEEK?

The experience of Hell Week is what SEALs draw from when situations are cold, dark, and miserable. It proves to all SEALs that the human body can do ten times the amount of work and endure ten times the amount of pain and discomfort than the average human thinks possible. SEALs learn how to remain calm and react properly in hostile situations; how to persevere in the face of adversity; and most importantly, they learn the value of teamwork. The last three weeks of First Phase are spent learning hydrographic reconnaissance and recuperating a little from your 120-hour personal test. Rarely do men quit after Hell Week.

SECOND PHASE (DIVING)

Diving Phase lasts for seven weeks. During this period, physical training continues and the workouts get harder. Students have to run their four-mile runs a minute faster, swim their two-mile swims five minutes faster, and decrease their obstacle course each week of Second Phase. On top of the progressively difficult physical training, the number one priority of Second Phase is teaching students SCUBA (Self Contained Underwater Breathing Apparatus) diving. Students are taught two types of SCUBA: open circuit (compressed air) and closed circuit (100% oxygen rebreather). After Second Phase, students will be basic combat divers, with the physical ability to insert miles from a target and conduct several types of missions. This skill separates SEALs from all other Special Operations Forces.

THIRD PHASE (LAND WARFARE)

Third Phase lasts for nine weeks. Demolitions, reconnaissance, and land warfare are the number-one priorities of this phase; however, this is also the most physically demanding phase of the three. Ten-mile runs, four-mile swims, and hundreds of pushups, pullups and situps must be done several times a week. Skills such as land navigation, small arms handling, small-unit tactics, patrolling techniques, rappelling, and military explosives are also mastered. This training is held at San Clemente Island and is classified. You'll have to get there before you learn any more about the highly physical and technical training of BUD/S Third Phase.

RUNNING AT BUD/S

To most BUD/S students, running is the most physically and mentally challenging exercise they will face. It is extremely important to have a strong running base before you arrive at BUD/S. If you do not, you will be one of the majority who become injured during the First Phase, and will have a greater chance of being dropped from the BUD/S program. Running up to four or five times a week at least three months prior to arriving at BUD/S is absolutely necessary. Chapter Five is devoted to teaching the proper techniques of running in the sand and preventing common overuse injuries.

PT AT BUD/S

Upper body strength is a must at BUD/S. BUD/S PT lasts at least two hours and is conducted 3–4 times a week. These workouts can test even the seasoned athlete. TRUST ME; DON'T GO TO BUD/S IF YOU HAVE NEVER DONE THE EXERCISES IN THIS BOOK! You should be able to do several hundred pushups, situps, and flutter kicks in a complete workout. Practice these NOW, before you get to BUD/S.

WARNING: Some of these exercises (flutter kicks, leg levers, abdominal stretches…) have been proven and disproven in certain studies to be harmful to your lower back. Navy SEALs have been performing these exercises for over 30 years. Former SEALs in their fifties and sixties still perform these exercises—but do these exercises at your own risk!

SWIMMING AT BUD/S

You will have two-mile timed ocean swims wearing fins every week at BUD/S. It is an absolute necessity to swim with fins prior to arriving at BUD/S. You have to strengthen your ankles and hip flexors by swimming with fins. There is no other way to prepare yourself, and the swimming will be extra challenging for you if you are not prepared. However, the biggest challenge to all BUD/S students is the water temperature—70 degrees in the summer, 55 degrees in the winter. It does not take long to become hypothermic in temperatures this cold. Ask any SEAL and he will tell you that getting used to being cold was the hardest part of BUD/S. Most of the students who quit say they do so because the water was too cold for them.

BUD/S OBSTACLE COURSE

The BUD/S "O-Course" is a test of upper body strength and cardiovascular stamina. The only way to improve at the O-Course is by constantly practicing. It will help if you climb ropes and do hundreds of pullups prior to arriving at BUD/S. Obstacles with ropes surrounded by soft sand will challenge anyone, but it will break a person who has slacked off on his upper body exercises. Climb ropes as often as you run—four to five times per week!

FINAL COMMENTS ABOUT BUD/S

BUD/S is said to be the "toughest military training in the world." It is definitely challenging both mentally and physically. The instructors at BUD/S will make demands on your body for six months. You must be in the best shape of your life to succeed at BUD/S; but more importantly, you must be mentally focused and strong or you will become one of the 70–75% who drop out of training. The workout I designed will make you physically fit. If you have the desire to stick to this workout every day, by the end you might just have what it takes to succeed at BUD/S. You will definitely be physically prepared, but will you be mentally prepared? That is up to you.

This is what you must prepare yourself for:

First Phase	Second Phase	Third Phase
four-mile timed runs	four-mile timed runs	four-mile timed runs
up to one-mile swims	up to two-mile ocean swims	up to three-mile ocean swims
obstacle courses	obstacle courses	obstacle courses
50m underwater swim	5.5-mile ocean swim*	15-mile timed run*
upper body PT	upper body PT	upper body PT
soft-sand runs	soft-sand runs	soft-sand runs
HELLWEEK*		

*Special one-time events. All other events occur WEEKLY!

HOW DO YOU MENTALLY PREPARE YOURSELF FOR BUD/S?

First, being physically prepared will help you become mentally tough. Just as your endurance will grow each day with this program, so will your confidence. Knowing in your heart that you can complete the evolutions listed above without even thinking of quitting is the secret to excelling at BUD/S. For me, knowing that if I quit, I had to serve on a ship for the next five years was enough motivation. Others have something to prove to themselves, their family, or their friends. The key is to find what motivates you to succeed and then stay focused on that motivator when the days are long and the nights are just beginning. During Hell Week, take one hour at a time. Do not think that because you are exhausted and are only two hours into the 120-hour week that you cannot complete Hell Week. Instead think about making it to the next meal. Students get to sit, rest, and eat for almost an hour every six hours during Hell Week.

COLD WATER

It will help if you become accustomed to ocean water, especially water temperature in the 60s. Ocean swims and body surfing are great ways to prepare yourself for the "Surf Zone." If you do not have access to ocean water, swim with fins in a pool for a couple of hours a few times a week. You have to realize that the BUD/S instructors can only keep you in the water for a certain period of time—NOTHING WILL LAST FOREVER.

SAFETY!

I do not recommend swimming alone in a pool, but especially not in the ocean. Navy SEALs always have a "swim buddy" with them no mater what they are doing. If you do not have a friend who shares your same desires and work ethic, at least have a lifeguard watch you swim.

Good luck—I hope you find what motivates you to never quit!

EQUIPMENT AND FACILITIES NEEDED FOR THIS WORKOUT:

- Access to a pool, either 25m or 25 yd, 50m or 50 yd.
- Access to a track or measured running area, 400m/400 yd.
- Access to pullup bars and dip bars (parallel bars).

NUTRITION

AN OVERALL DIET FOR BURNING FAT AND GETTING LEAN

Contributed by Jud Dean
B.S. in Nutrition/Dietetics
University of Delaware

By purchasing this book, you have entered an action stage. It shows you are serious about weight loss and changing your life. Now that you have spent money, you have committed yourself, at least financially, to starting your healthy lifestyle. Would you waste your money and just have this book collect dust?

It's time to begin your investment in your future, an investment that will pay out later in life when you have far fewer heath problems than your peers. Now, let's talk about your diet and how it can help you reach your goals.

Nutrition

HOW TO EAT

The biggest problem most of us have is not knowing about proper nutrition. It may come as a surprise to know that 3 square meals a day is not the best way to eat. Even if it was, most of us only eat 2 large meals a day anyway.

The real way to lose weight is to consume multiple meals over the course of the day. Ten percent of the calories you burn during the day come from consuming food, whether from chewing and swallowing, or from digesting. What logically follows is that the more often you eat, the more your body has to work, which will increase your metabolism and help you burn fat.

Ideally, you should try to eat 5 to 6 meals a day. These should not be large meals or "wow I am stuffed" meals. Your goal should be to eat enough to get you to your next small meal, in roughly 3 hours (this is how long it takes for the stomach to completely empty).

You must have an understanding of portion control. Many restaurants serve 3 to 4 times an actual serving size. For example, a serving of meat is the size of a deck of playing cards. When you eat out, instead of clearing your plate bring some home with you for meals the following day.

Balancing the food groups is another frequent problem. When you make your meals at home, try splitting your plate into three parts (first in half, and then one of those in half). Your plate will have three sections; two smaller sections and one larger section. Vegetables or fruits should fill the large area, and meat and carbohydrates in the two smaller areas. You will cut down dramatically on calories and fat.

WHAT TO EAT

There are three major areas of macronutrients: protein, carbohydrates, and fat. All of them are necessary to build muscles and to keep your body running. The best thing for you to do when dieting is to finetune how much of each nutrient you eat.

Protein

Proteins are the muscle's food. Your body takes amino acids from digested proteins and uses them for muscle repair. There are two different categories of proteins:

- whey (the one found in most shakes and supplements)
- casein (found in milks)

It is essential that you consume both these types of protein. You will want to consume the whey proteins, which are in egg whites, fish, and protein powders, early in the morning or after a workout. Whey is the Ferrari of protein; it gets in the blood stream quickly after a workout. Your body will need this quick hit so it can repair your muscles immediately. Likewise, as soon as you wake up, it's important to have some whey protein. After all, your body has been using nutrients all night and needs a quick fix to start muscle repair, growth, and activate your metabolism.

Casein is slowly digested. It may take a while to get into the bloodstream, but it gets the job done every time. This protein should be consumed in the middle of the day, so your body gets a constant supply of protein all day long. It is found in foods such as red meat, poultry, and whole eggs. Remember, even though protein is not as bad as fat, it can still make you fat. Eating anything in excess will make you fat, because it will cause excess calories.

PROTEIN	
Unhealthy	**Healthy**
fried chicken	chicken breast—no skin
hamburger	ground turkey breast
cheese	non-fat cheese
fatty steak	deer steak
2% milk	skim milk
tuna and mayo	tuna and honey mustard

Carbohydrates

Carbohydrates have been getting bad publicity over the past few years thanks to the Atkins diet and many other fad diets. However, this is a tough workout plan and you better get your carbs or else you are going to be in deep trouble. Carbs are the energy builders within your body. Without enough carbohydrates, you are going to feel very lazy and will not have enough energy to complete the workouts. Carbohydrates are also essential to help your body absorb protein, which, as discussed, helps the muscles grow and repair.

The amount of carbs that you will consume is dependent on how hard you are going to be training, but a good starting point to consider is 2 grams per pound of your body weight, per day. So, for example, if you weigh 200 pounds you should consume 400 grams of carbohydrates on a daily basis. Remember, as your weight loss progresses, change your carbohydrate intake accordingly. Excess calories will be what is going to make you fat.

CARBOHYRATES	
Unhealthy	**Healthy**
white bread	wheat bread
white pasta	wheat pasta
white rice	brown rice
white potato	sweet potato/yam
boiled vegetables	steamed vegetables

Fats

Now for what everyone thinks is scary: fat. The Dietary Guidelines suggest a diet between 20–35% fat, and the guidelines here are on the lower end of this scale. The different types of fats are:

- monounsaturated fats
- saturated fats
- polyunsaturated fats
- trans fats

Monounsaturated fates are the healthiest fats. Our body needs a certain amount for survival, and these are what are referred to when you hear people discussing "good fats." Monounsaturated fats are found in products such as olive oil and nuts.

The other types of fats should be consumed in very small amounts. Saturated fats are found in your cookies and chips, polyunsaturated fats in your salad dressings and mayo, and trans fats can be found in your pastries and candies.

To keep a low-fat diet, find alternatives to the fats you are consuming. For example, instead of eating butter, use Smart Balance spray. Instead of mayo, use honey mustard, or find a no-fat mayo. The best option in any diet is to eat the healthiest choices you can find.

FATS	
Unhealthy	**Healthy**
vegetable shortening	nut, canola, olive oils; salmon and fish oils
hard stick margarine	corn, soy, safflower, and sunflower oils

DRINK LOTS OF WATER

Many people do not drink enough water. It's often possible to think that you are hungry when you are actually thirsty.

Water is crucial as it is a key factor in almost every function and reaction of your body. If you drink enough water, your body will burn stored fat for energy. As an added bonus, if the water is cold your body will burn fat by trying to warm it up. I consume far more water than the recommended 8 glasses or 64 ounces. With the rigorous workout that follows, it's recommended to drink one 32-ounce Gatorade (half before workout and half after), along with four 32-ounce bottles of water sipped on throughout the day. If you feel dehydrated drink more. If your urine is not clear drink more.

Water will also help to curb your appetite if you drink two glasses 15 minutes prior to eating. Drink water to fill your stomach, because you will eat less.

PRE-WORKOUT MEALS

Before Cardio Workout
(running, swimming, biking at medium to high intensity for 30 to 40 minutes)
Carbohydrates 75% to 100% / Protein 25% to 0%

- Eat a small snack to boost sugar levels in your body especially if your workout is before your morning meal.

- For a boost after not eating for 10 to 12 hours, try fruit or fruit juice 20 minutes prior to the workout.

- Small amounts of protein can be eaten pre-workout and will help your post-workout recovery if your workout lasts longer than 40 minutes.

- Good pre-workout snacks include bananas, apples, oranges, carrots, juice, and Gatorade.

- 1 to 2 hours before exercising, try yogurt, a protein drink, milk, boiled egg, a slice of meat or cheese, or a Slimfast meal replacement bar.

- Sip water and a carbohydrate drink throughout the workout.

Before Lifting or Calisthenics
(1 to 2 hours prior to lifting)
Carbohydrates 75% / Protein 25%

- Eat protein foods and carbohydrates before working out so you replace the glycogen stores and will give you a needed protein boost post-workout.

- After you work out, eat protein and carbohydrates and minimize your fatty foods.

- Good pre-workout snacks are bananas, berries, boiled eggs, and tuna fish.

- Protein and carbohydrate sources include tuna, chicken, boiled eggs, and green leafy salads with tomatoes, broccoli, cucumber, carrots, onions, and light dressing or oil.

- Protein or carb replacement drinks are great if post workout occurs mid-day or early morning.

POST-WORKOUT MEALS

- To replace carbohydrates and electrolytes lost during the workout, drink Powerade or Gatorade immediately after working out.

- Add protein to help rebuild muscles within 30 minutes of working out.

ONE WEEK BEFORE A PST

While your workouts taper down the week before your PST, your nutrition should not. There is a big difference between having an off day and a rest day. On a rest day, you do not work out, but your diet stays the same.

During the week before the PST, you want to eat foods that will give you the energy you need to do well on test day. We discussed your pre-workout meal, and that is the kind of meal you should eat the morning of your PST. You don't want your body to have to deal with anything new or different on test day. Your body should think it is business as usual.

If your test day is Saturday morning, you should start drinking more water than usual on Tuesday, straight through until test day.

On Wednesday night, you should have a meal of pasta. (I like to make angel hair, ground turkey breast, non-fat marinara sauce, and 3 bell peppers.) This will be your meals for Thursday afternoon, night, and Friday afternoon. This carb-loading will give you the extra energy you need on Saturday. You may get tired of the pasta, but eat it until it is completely gone. It normally takes me about 5 meals to complete the batch; three meals on Thursday, and two on Friday.

Remember to consume a lot of fluid this week. I like to drink a Gatorade prior to bed on these nights so that my body has extra fluid and electrolytes while I sleep. You will get tired of waking up to use the restroom, but it will all be worth it come Saturday afternoon when you are getting your best score ever.

I also recommend trying this a few times before your test day: Set aside a Saturday a few weeks before your test to have a practice run to see how your body feels. This way you can make changes that will fit your personal body type. Nutrition works different with different individuals, so you may have to change a thing here or there to give yourself the best chance at success.

WEEKENDS

Do not think the weekends are a free time to eat and act however you want. According to the *Journal of Obesity Research*, Americans consume an extra 115 calories per day on the weekends. This means that with 104 weekend days a year, that those extra calories will give you an extra 3.5 pounds a year. Be smart and do not sabotage your weekday efforts with carefree weekends.

DEHYDRATION

It is easy to design a dehydration diet that results in losing 10 pounds of water weight within several days. Many people are encouraged by these rapid results. But be wary: dehydrating your body and losing 2–3% of your body weight can result in a 7% drop in your physical performance. Your body is over 75% water and needs around this percentage in order to function properly.

Sweat is not just water, but also contains salt and electrolytes. These compounds help regulate nerve and muscular function. Without them, entire systems start to break down and this can be fatal. Once you stop sweating, there is no mechanism in your body to regulate body temperature and you could overheat and die from heat stroke.

Removing additional water from your digestive system by diuretics and laxatives causes the kidneys to overwork and eventually stop functioning. When this occurs, the liver assists the body in excretion waste products (if it can) and it stops with its primary mission of metabolizing fat as an energy source. So in a nutshell, doing this will shut down your entire metabolism as your body tries desperately to cling onto any remaining water and fat. This can actually cause the opposite to your desires—your body now is retaining water and fat just to survive.

This process is a vicious cycle. The true way to burn fat and lose weight for the long term is to actually drink water plus exercise. I drink over a gallon of water a day but I also exercise for more than two hours a day usually. I would recommend 2–3 quarts for women and 3–4 quarts for men per day of water to see huge results in weight loss. The equation looks like this:

Fat loss = water + oxygen (from cardiovascular exercise)

Safe weight loss is around from 2–3 pounds per week (using this formula). Losing any more weight than this and you are losing water weight—which will return as quickly as it left.

If you lose weight too quickly, much of the weight loss will be from muscle tissue. It is estimated that when people lose over 2 pounds of weight a week, 30–40% of the weight lost will be muscle. This is a disaster for keeping the weight off in the long term because muscle is five times more active metabolically than fat tissue.

EXERCISE AND HEALTHY EATING IS THE FIRST PRIORITY

The aim of an exercise program is to lose fat—without losing your muscle mass and without reducing your metabolic rate. In order to do this, the exercise program needs to be customized to your fitness level and the specific goal of fat loss.

Good nutrition is very important for fat loss, and focusing on health and health-promoting foods is far more productive than focusing on fat loss and denial of favorite foods. Adopt a whole food diet, avoid salt, fat, sugar, additives, preservatives, processed and refined foods, for this lifestyle change. By increasing intake of natural foods with high fiber and water content (fruit and vegetables), more food can be eaten to appease the appetite without gaining weight.

A whole food diet also has a much higher vitamin and mineral content than a typical diet containing processed and refined foods. Dieting is such a negative term. Think of this as "eating to lose weight."

Together, aerobic exercise and resistance training are the ideal combination to achieve your goal fat loss.

STRETCHING

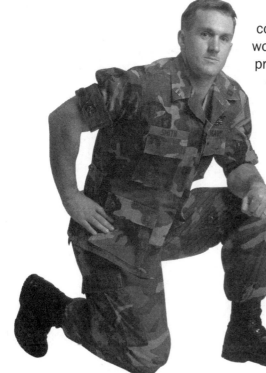

The following stretches should be completed before and after every workout. Stretching will minimize or prevent the onset of muscle soreness due to rigorous physical activity. It only takes a few minutes to stretch (preferably 10 minutes before the workout and 10–15 minutes after you are finished). If you consistently stretch, you will minimize your risk of injuries, your muscles will feel less sore, and your flexibility will increase, thus helping to make you a faster swimmer and runner.

PRE/POST WORKOUT STRETCHING ROUTINE

Stretches	Repetitions/Time
Jog	1/4 mile
Neck rotations	30 sec.
Arm and Shoulder	30 sec. each arm
Arm Circles	1 min.
Chest	30 sec.
Abdominal	30 sec.
Lower Back	30 sec.
Groin Stretch	30 sec.
ITB	30 sec. each leg
Thighs	30 sec. each leg.
Toe Touches	30 sec.
Calves	30 sec. each leg
Hamstring	30 sec.
Jumping Jacks	25 (4-count)

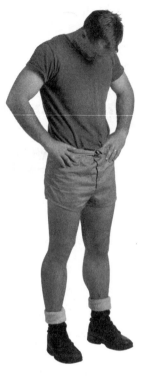

FRONT TO BACK

Relax your neck muscles and move your head slowly up and down. Try to touch your chin to your chest on the down movement. Continue for 30 seconds.

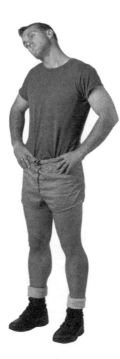

Be careful with neck stretches and do not go too far back or to the side. Just stretch the muscles of the neck by moving gingerly through a natural range of motion.

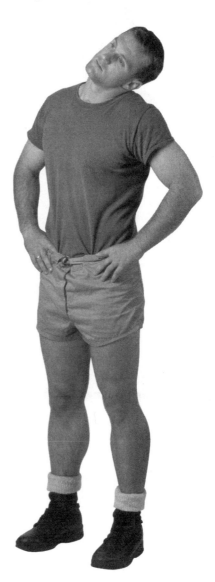

SIDE TO SIDE

Relax your neck muscles and move your head slowly to the left and right. Move your head as if you were trying to touch your shoulder to your ear. Continue for 30 seconds.

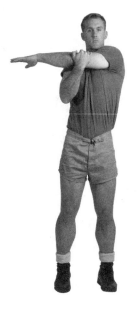

ARM AND SHOULDER STRETCH #1

With your left hand, grab your fight arm at the elbow and pull across your body. Hold for 15 seconds— switch arms.

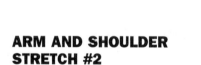

ARM AND SHOULDER STRETCH #2

Extend your arms over your head. With your left hand, grab your right arm at the elbow. Pull arm toward your head and lean with the pull, stretching the arm, shoulder, and back. Hold for 15 seconds—switch arms.

Arm Circles

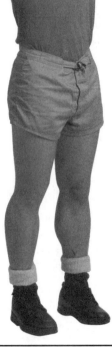

SIDE CIRCLES

Extend your arms out to both sides. Rotate your arms in small circles forward and backward. Continue for 30 seconds each direction.

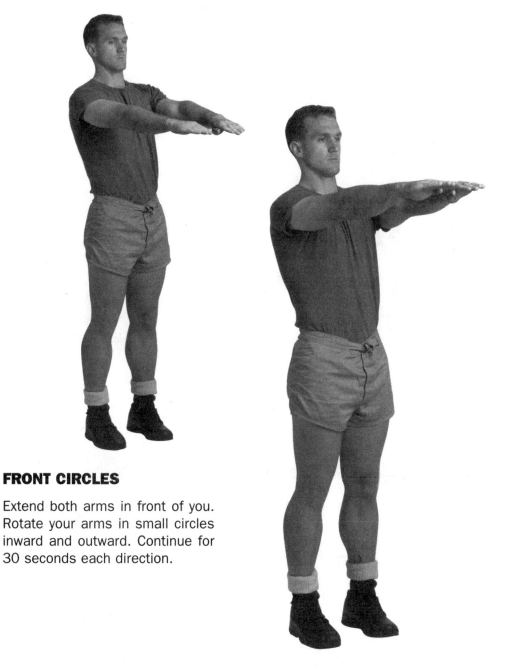

FRONT CIRCLES

Extend both arms in front of you.
Rotate your arms in small circles
inward and outward. Continue for
30 seconds each direction.

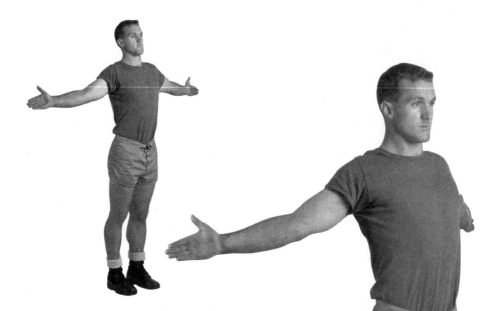

CHEST STRETCH #1

With arms extended on both sides of your body about shoulder height, slowly press arms backward. Keep back straight and chest bowed. Hold for 30 seconds.

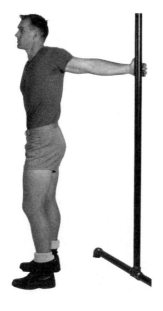

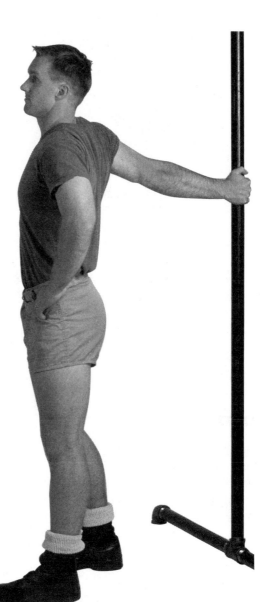

WALL STRETCH

Place right arm on wall about shoulder height. Turn body away from the wall to the left. Hold arm in place. Hold for 15 seconds. Switch and repeat.

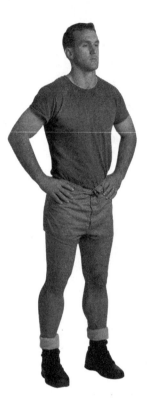

STANDING

With your hands on your waist, slowly lean backward by pushing your hips forward and slightly arching your back. Hold for 15 seconds—repeat.

SNAKES

Lay on your stomach. Place elbows under your chest and slowly lift your head and shoulders up, stretching your abdominal muscles. Hold for 15 seconds—repeat.

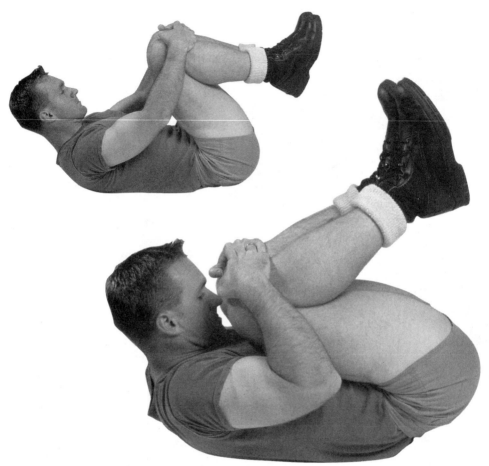

CHEST TO KNEES

Lay on your back. Bring your knees to your chest and your head toward your knees. Hold for 15 seconds.

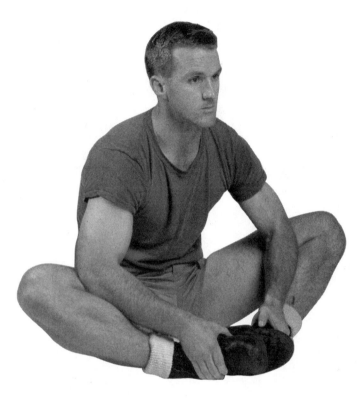

BUTTERFLY

Sit on the floor with both legs bent outward and the soles of your feet touching each other. Grab your ankles with your hands and push down on your thighs with your elbows. Hold for 15 seconds—repeat.

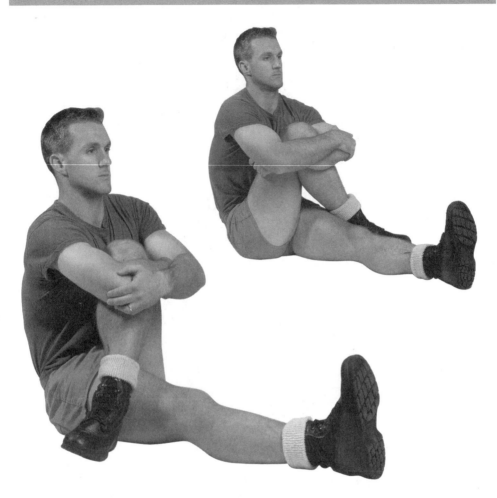

ITB STRETCH #1 (ILIO TIBIAL BAND)

Sit on the floor with both legs extended in front of you. Cross your right leg over your left. Bend and pull right leg to your chest and hold for 15 seconds. Switch and repeat.*

*Author's Note: Injury to the ITB due to overuse is very common among BUD/S students. For this reason, injury to the ITB is sometimes referred to as "I Tried BUD/S."

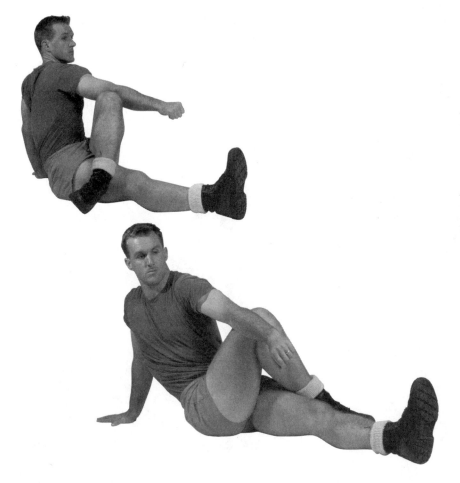

ITB STRETCH #2

In the same position as Stretch #1, twist to the side of bent leg to stretch your lower back and ITB. Try to look in the opposite direction of your feet. Hold for 15 seconds. Switch and repeat.

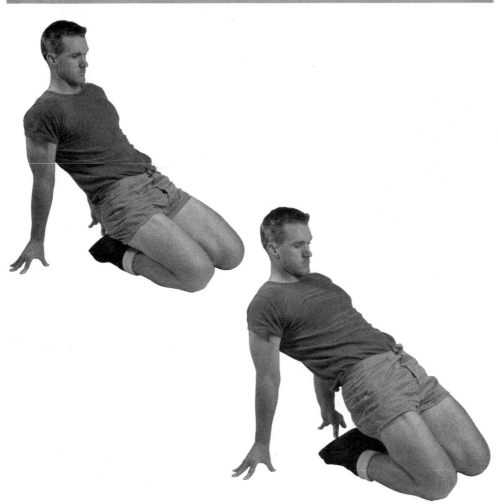

SITTING

Sit on your knees and heels. Lean backward so you can touch the floor behind you. Push your hips upward and hold for 15 seconds—repeat.

STANDING

Stand on your left leg. Grab your right foot behind you and pull it to your buttocks. Try to keep both knees together. Hold for 15 seconds. Switch and repeat.

Toe Touchers

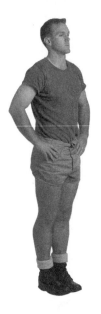

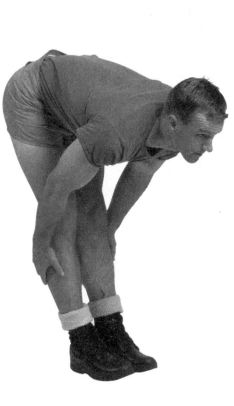

STANDING OR SITTING

With your feet together, bend at the waist and grab the back of your calves with both hands. Hold for 15 seconds—repeat.

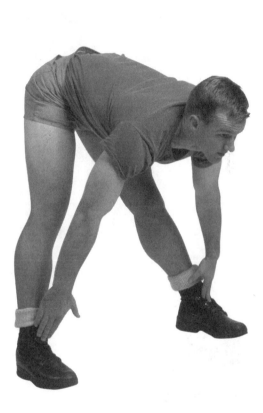

STANDING OR SITTING

With feet spread apart, bend at the waist and hold your back flat, stretching your hamstrings and lower back. Hold for 15 seconds—repeat.

Calf Stretches

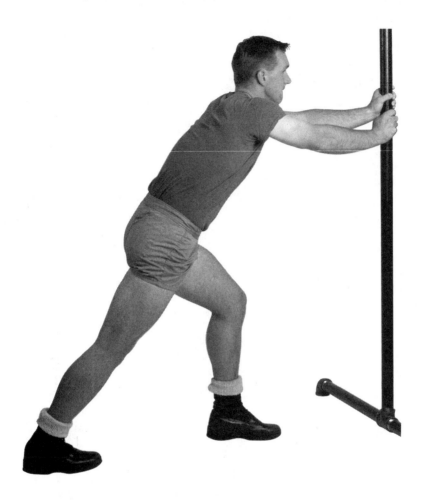

GASTROCNEMIUS

Stand about four feet away from a wall or other sturdy object. With most of your weight on one leg, keep that leg straight and lean into the wall. Hold for 15 seconds—switch legs and repeat.

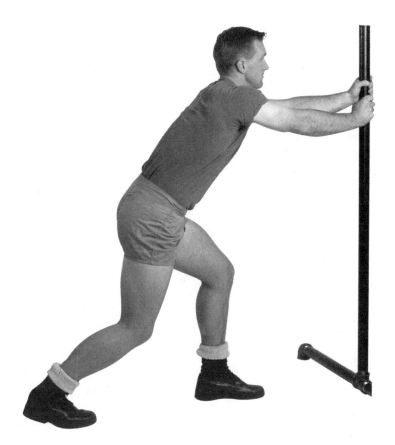

SOLEUS

Same stance as the Gastrocnemius Stretch, but bend your back knee slightly. You will feel the stretch in your Achilles tendon. Hold for 15 seconds—switch and repeat.

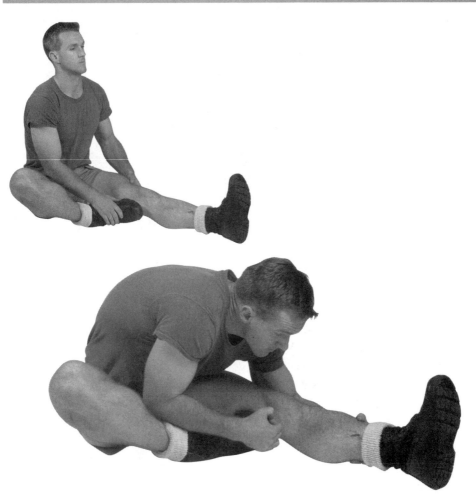

HURDLER STRIDE

Sit on the floor with legs extended in front of you. Bend right knee and place the sole of your right foot against the inside of your left knee. Grab feet and hold stretch for 15 seconds. Switch and repeat.

WARMUP

Standing with hands by your side and feet together, jump and spread your legs while simultaneously placing your arms over your head. Repeat for one minute.

PHYSICAL TRAINING

Physical Training, or PT, is a series of calisthenics and other exercises which are designed to strengthen your body. A combination of these exercises is referred to as "grinder PT" at BUD/S.

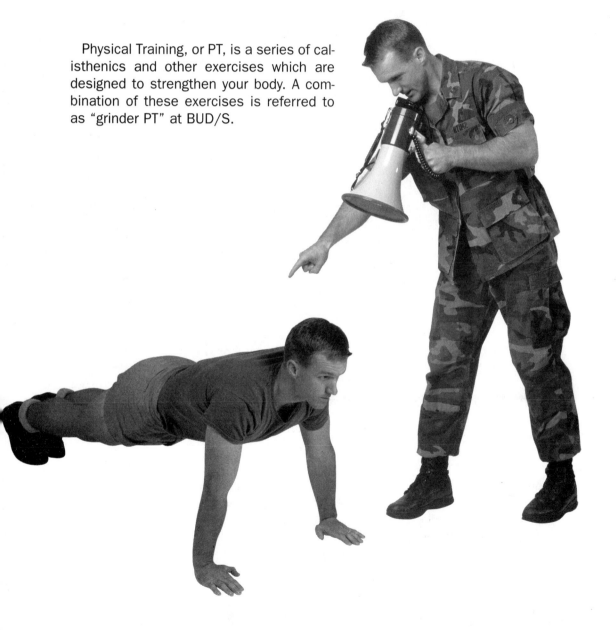

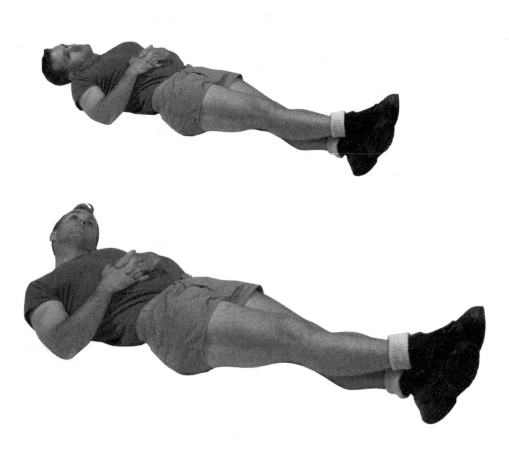

NECK EXERCISE #1: SIDE TO SIDE

Lay on your back. Lift your head off the floor and move it from side to side for specified number of repetitions.*

*Author's Note: The number of repetitions for each exercise will vary depending on which day of which week of the program you are completing (see the 12 Weeks to BUD/S Workout chapter beginning on page 155). For example, in Week One, you will do 20 repetitions of the side-to-side neck exercise shown above. In Week Ten, you will do 100 repetitions of this exercise.

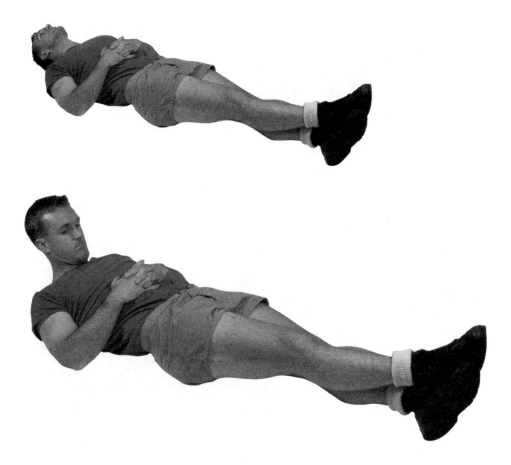

NECK EXERCISE #2: UP AND DOWN

Lay on your back. Lift your head off the floor and move it up and down for specified number of repetitions.

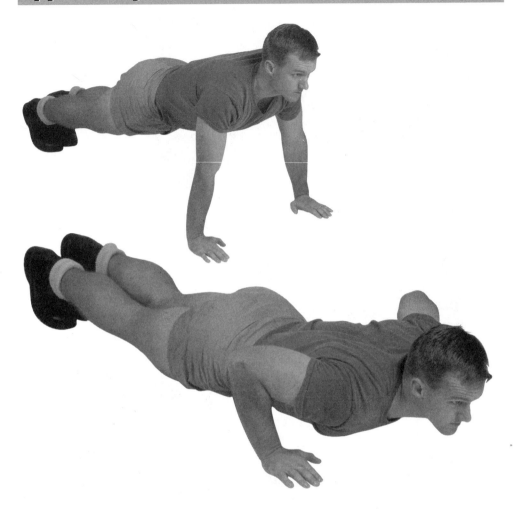

PUSHUPS: REGULAR

With hands at shoulder width, place your palms on the ground, keeping your feet together and back straight. Push your body up until your arms are straight. Touch chest to ground each repetition.

Pushups are a great punishment exercise. For the programs in this book, you will be required to perform pushups several days in a row. This goes against every physiology rule of good training, but that is the nature of the beast in these types of military training environments. You will also be required to remain in the leaning rest for many minutes at a time. It is smart to shake out your shoulders occasionally and stretch after a long "rest."

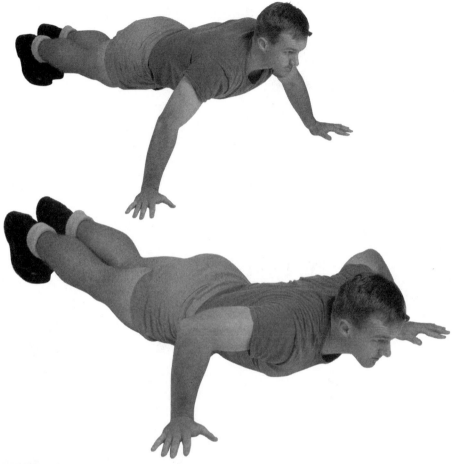

PUSHUPS: WIDE

With hands wider than shoulder width, place your palms on the ground, keeping feet together and back straight. Push your body up until your arms are straight. Touch chest to ground each repetition.

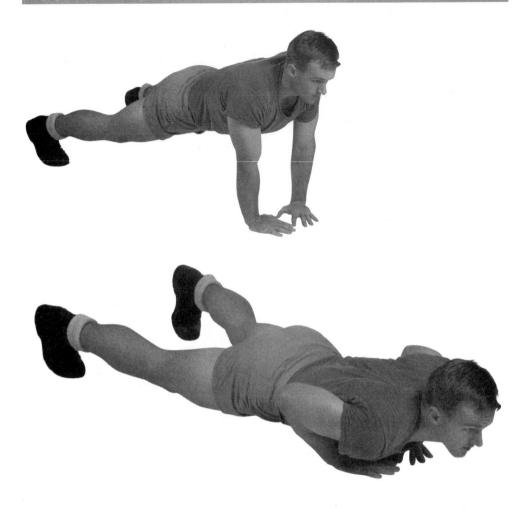

PUSHUPS: TRICEPS

With hands touching, forming a tri-angle with your index fingers and thumbs meeting (as shown above), place palms on the ground, spreading your legs and keeping your back straight. Push your body up until your arms are straight. Touch chest to hands each repetition.

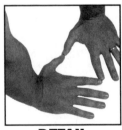

DETAIL

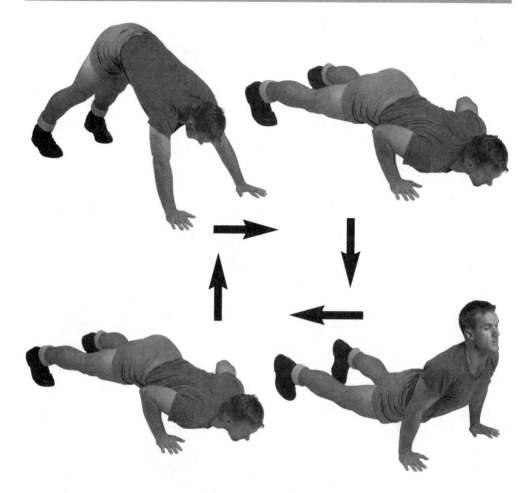

PUSHUPS: DIVE BOMBERS

Get into the pushup position, but bend at the waist and stick your buttocks in the air (Figure 1). Keeping your buttocks in the air, place chest to the ground in between your hands (Figure 2). Continue forward movement and push your chest through your hands and up by straightening your arms (Figure 3). Reverse the process and return back to starting position (Figure 4).

2

1

3

4

5

PUSHUPS: 8-COUNT BODY BUILDERS

These should be done in quick succession.

6

1. Full Squat.
2. Leg Thrust.
3. Pushup down.
4. Pushup up.
5. Spread legs.
6. Close legs.
7. Reverse leg thrust.
8. Standing.

7

8

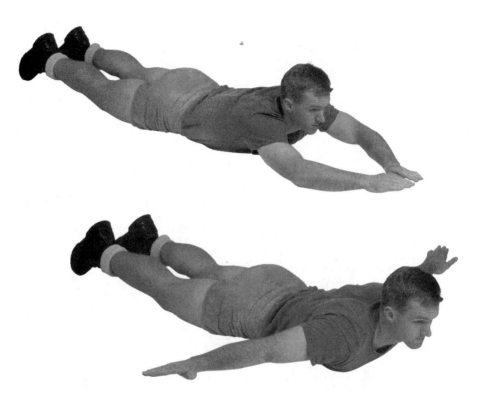

ARM HAULERS

Lay on your stomach with your back arched slightly. Move your arms from the starting position over your head to your side (as if you were swimming). Keep your feet off the ground as well. This exercise works shoulders, lower back, and buttocks.

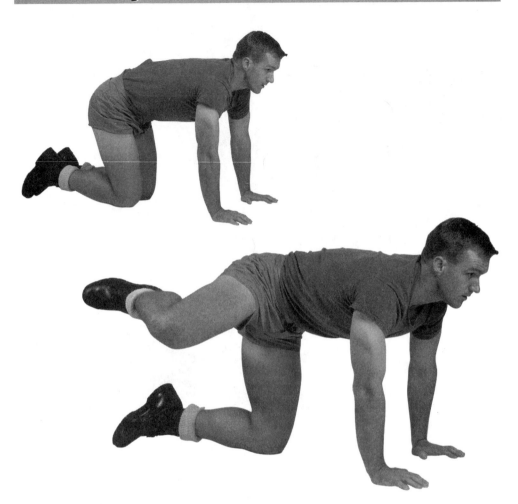

DIRTY DOGS

Get into the "all fours" position. Lift your leg from your hip joint to the side for the specified number of repetitions. You may drop to your elbows for more comfort on your lower back. Switch sides and repeat.

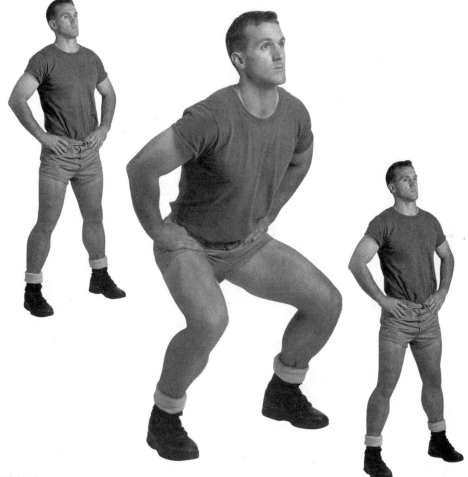

SQUATS

With feet about shoulder width apart, back straight, and eyes looking up, lower yourself by bending your legs almost 90 degrees at the knees. Slowly raise yourself after you have reached almost 90 degrees.

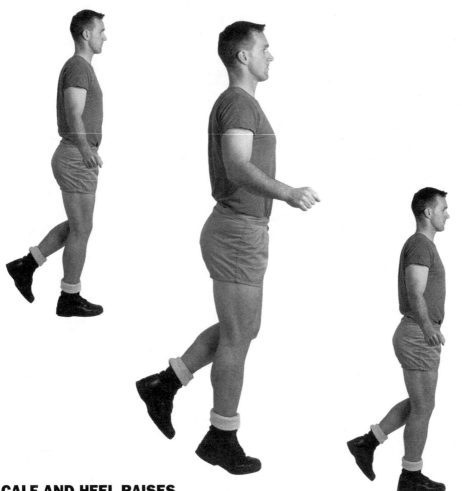

CALF AND HEEL RAISES

Stand on one leg. Lift yourself up onto the balls of your feet by flexing the ankle joint and calf muscle. Switch legs and repeat for specified number of repetitions.

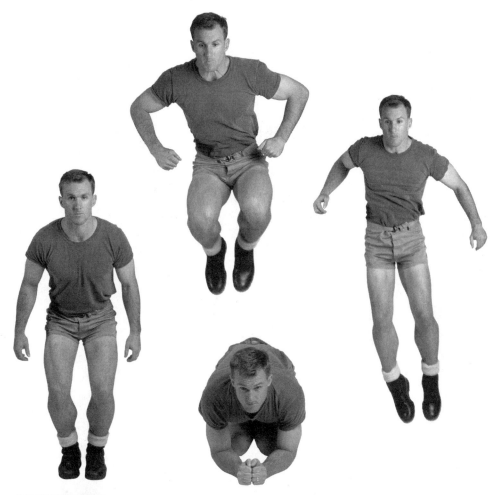

JUMPOVERS

Stand next to an object approximately 1.5–2 feet high. Jump from one side to the other for specified number of repetitions. Try to hit the ground on one side and jump back immediately after touching. Try not to double bounce.

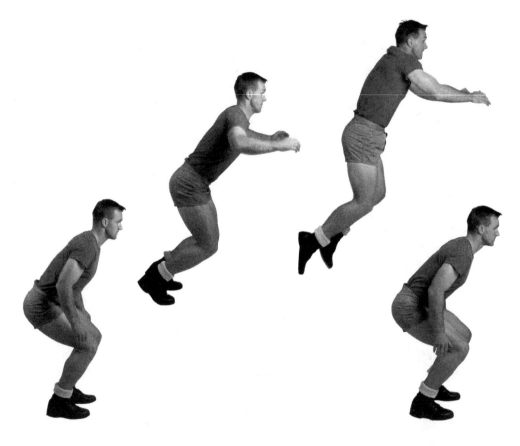

FROG HOPS

From the squatting position, jump forward as far as you can. Repeat for specified number of repetitions.

LUNGES

Take a big step forward with either leg. Lower your body by bending your knees and almost touching one knee to the floor. Switch legs and repeat.

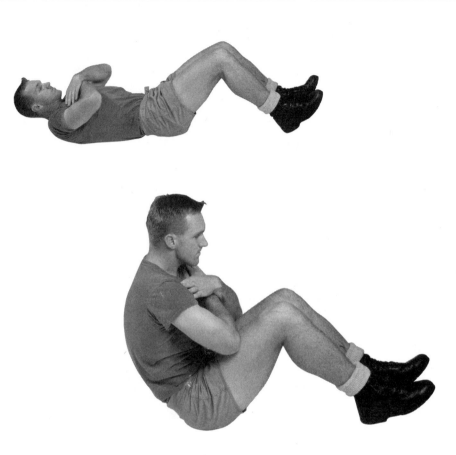

SITUPS: REGULAR

Lay on your back with your arms crossed over your chest and your knees slightly bent. Raise your upper body off the floor by contracting your stomach muscles. Touch your elbows to your thighs and repeat. Make sure you touch your shoulder blades to the floor each time.

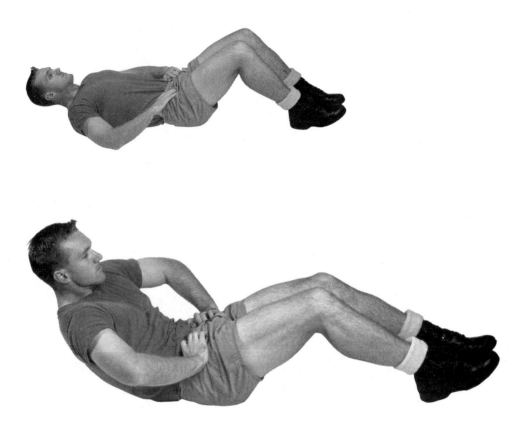

1/2 SITUP

Lay on your back and place your hands on your hips. Lift your upper body so your lower back just comes off the floor, then slowly let yourself back down to the starting position. Repeat for specified number of repetitions.

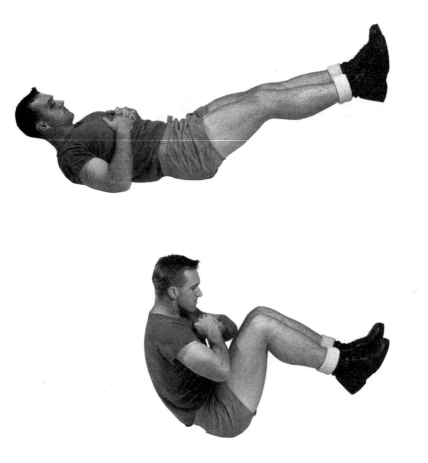

SITUPS: ATOMIC

Lay on your back. Lift your feet 6 inches off the floor and pull your knees toward your chest while simultaneously lifting your upper body off the floor.

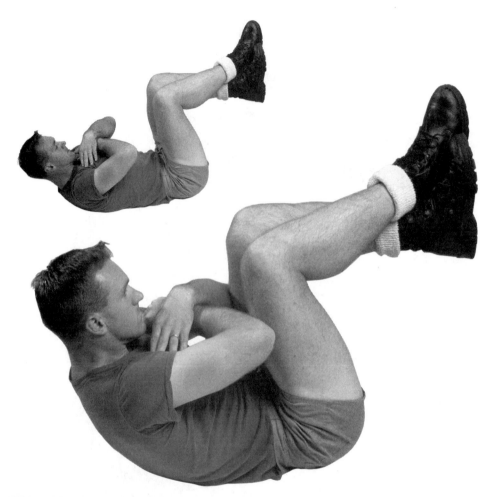

CRUNCHES: REGULAR

Lay on your back with your legs up in the air and bent at the knees, forming a 90 degree angle with your legs. Bring your elbows to your knees. DO NOT PUT YOUR HANDS BEHIND YOUR HEAD AND PULL ON YOUR NECK.

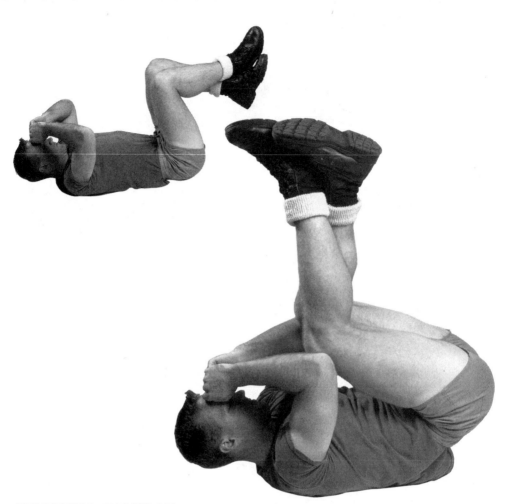

CRUNCHES: REVERSE

Lay on your back with your legs up in the air and bent at the knees, forming a 90 degree angle with your legs. Bring your knees to your elbows, lifting your lower back and buttocks off the ground. Keep your upper body still.

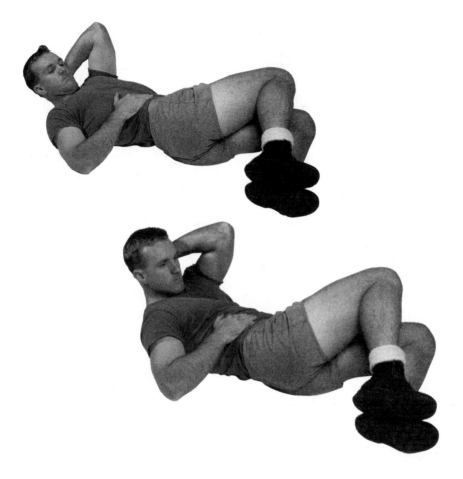

CRUNCHES: RIGHT

Lay with your shoulders and back flat on the floor, twisting your waist and legs so that you are laying on the left side of your hip. Crunch upward with your left arm and shoulder across your body toward the right side of your hip.

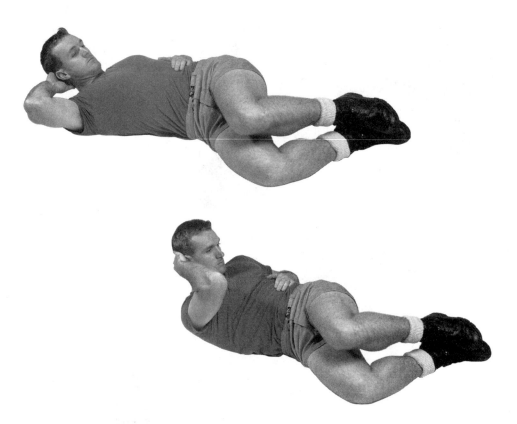

CRUNCHES: LEFT

Lay with your shoulders and back flat on the floor, twisting your waist and legs so that you are laying on the right side of your hip. Crunch upward with your right arm and shoulder across your body toward the left side of your hip.

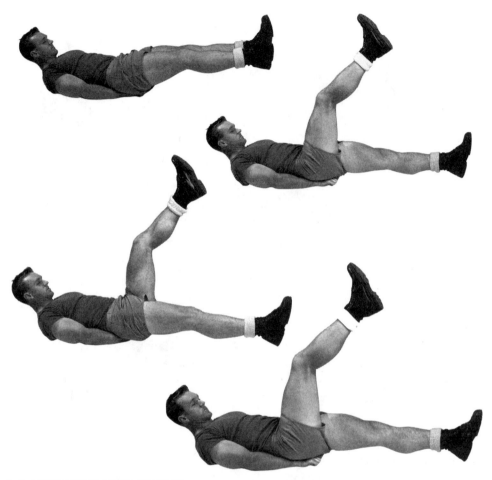

4-COUNT FLUTTER KICKS

Place your hands under your hips. Lift legs 6 inches off the ground and begin "walking," raising each leg approximately 3 feet off the ground. Keep your legs straight and constantly moving. With each "step" you take, count 1, so the sequence will go as follows: 1, 2, 3, 1; 1, 2, 3, 2; 1, 2, 3, 3; . . . for the specified number of repetitions.

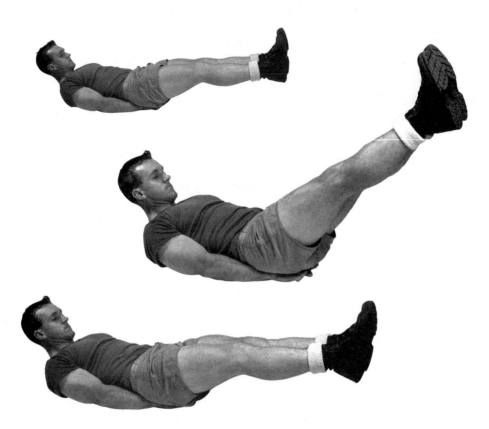

LEG LEVERS

Lay on your back with your hands under your hips and your legs together 6 inches off the floor. Lift your legs about 3 feet off the floor and slowly bring them down. Repeat. Do not let your legs touch the ground.

If you are looking to reduce strain on your lower back while performing the Leg Levers and 4-Count Flutter Kicks:

1) Lift your butt off of the ground by about an inch.
2) Place your hands underneath your butt bone, one on top of the other. This helps you to raise your butt higher, and takes some of the strain off the lower back.
3) Keep your knees straight and perform these exercises at the full range of motion of your hips. (Legs approximately six inches off of the floor vertically.)

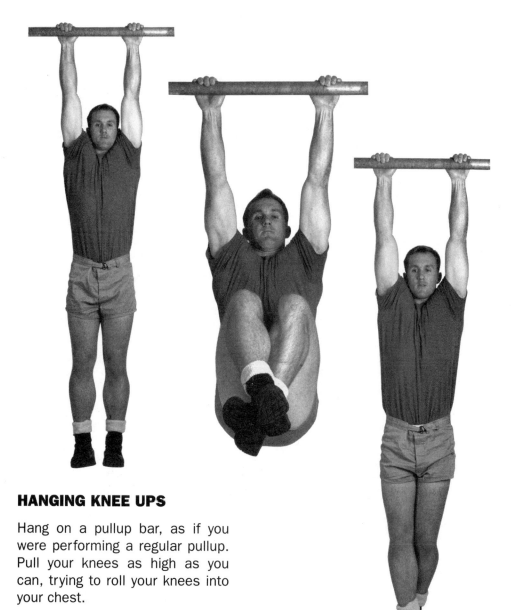

HANGING KNEE UPS

Hang on a pullup bar, as if you were performing a regular pullup. Pull your knees as high as you can, trying to roll your knees into your chest.

PULLUPS AND DIPS

There are five different types of pullups which work various groups of arm and back muscles. The pullup workout that requires sets of 2, 4, 6, 8, and 10 repetitions for every type of pullup is challenging, but offers moments of recovery and rest.

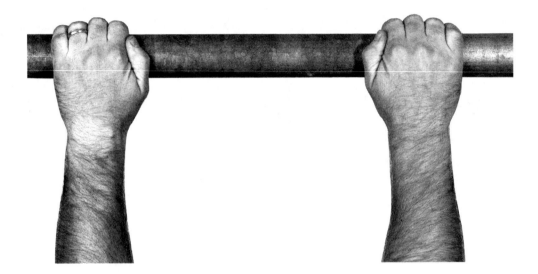

CORRECT GRIP

To strengthen your grip when doing pullups, make sure you use the correct grip shown above. This will increase the number of pullups you can do. Place your thumb next to your index finger and grip the bar with your fingers. Do not wrap your thumb around the bar.

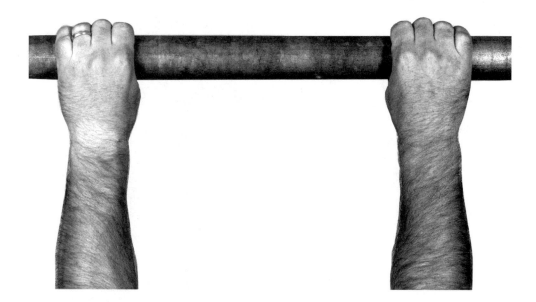

INCORRECT GRIP

The above photo, with thumbs and fingers wrapped around the bar, shows the grip that you should not use when doing pullups. With your thumb wrapped around the bar, your grip will weaken more quickly than if you use the proper grip shown on the opposite page.

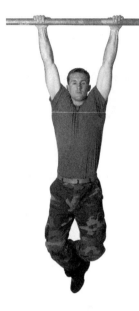

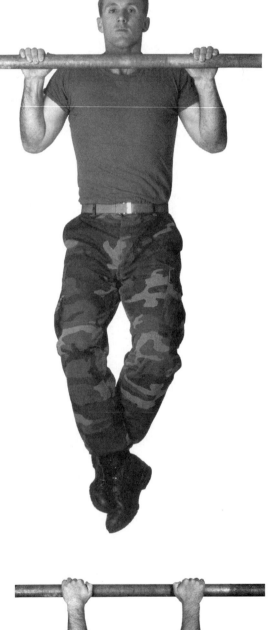

REGULAR GRIP

With hands at shoulder width (see below), grab the bar and pull yourself up so your chin is lifted above the bar. Hold yourself above the bar for one second and let yourself down in a slow, controlled manner.

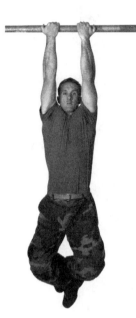

REVERSE GRIP

With your palms facing you (see below), grab the bar and pull your chin over the bar. Repeat for specified number of repetitions.

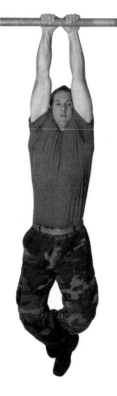

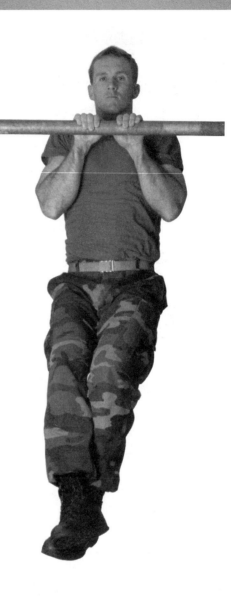

CLOSE GRIP

With your hands touching (or within 1 inch of each other), and palms facing away from you (see below), grab the bar and pull your chin over the bar. Repeat for specified number of repetitions.

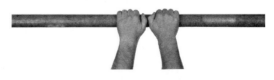

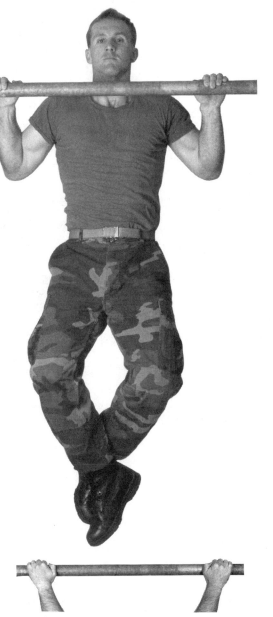

WIDE GRIP

With hands wider than shoulder width, and palms facing away from you (see below), grab the bar and pull your chin above it. Complete specified number of repetitions.

Pullups

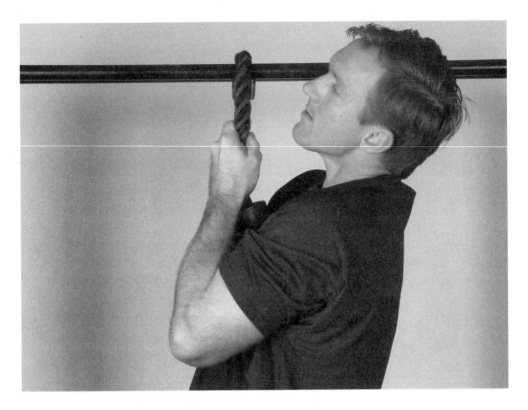

ROPE PULLUPS

Rope Pullups will prepare you for the obstacle course at SEAL Training.

You should perform pullups a maximum of three times a week—not every day. Every other day is recommended to allow you a chance to rest your back and arm muscles properly and prevent overtraining.

Never perform behind-the-neck pullups or pulldowns. These can cause shoulder impingement or other injuries of the rear shoulder and lower neck.

MORE PULLUP EXERCISES

The pullup is one of the most challenging exercises to perform. If you are overweight, especially if you are more than 10 pounds overweight, this can seriously affect your ability to do even a single pullups. But there is good news: The common denominator between men and women who can do pullups is that they practice them regularly. The best way to train to increase the number of pullups you can do is simply to do pullups every other day.

When you are burned out from doing pullups, or simply cannot do a negative or assisted version, start off with Bicep Curls and Bent-over Rows with Dumbbells.

Pullups are important for building the muscles needed for your profession. You will use them in the following places:

Over the wall or fence. The wall climb or jump in the obstacle course is challenging to people who lack upper body strength and the ability to coordinate a jump with an upper body pulling motion. The jump requires you getting your body high enough so that you are able to pull your torso on top of the wall.

Climbing rope or caving ladders. You will perform rope climbs and caving ladders over and over while doing your job. Whether it's climbing a fence or climbing up to a second story window using a caving ladder or rope, you can be better prepared for it if you practice rope or towel pullups.

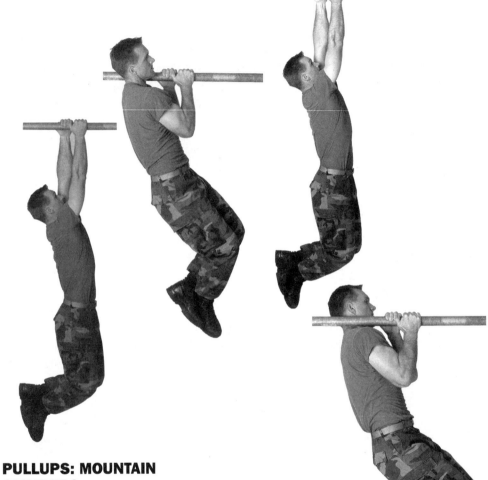

PULLUPS: MOUNTAIN CLIMBERS

Place your hands together on the bar, one palm facing you and the other facing away from you (see below). Pull yourself up and touch your shoulder to the bar. Repeat, pulling yourself up on the other side of the bar.

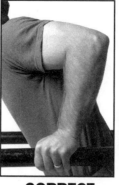 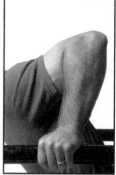

CORRECT   **INCORRECT**

BAR DIPS

Mount the two parallel bars with your hands on both sides of your body. Lift your body by straightening your arms. Do not lock your elbows. Slowly lower your body to a level where your arms make a 90 degree angle at the elbow joint. Do not go lower than 90 degrees, because this is bad for your shoulder joints.

RUNNING AT BUD/S

Running in sand is more difficult than running on pavement, but less stressful on your joints. After several weeks of running in sand, your leg muscles will become stronger and you will have more stamina than ever before. Running is also an excellent cross-training tool to increase leg muscle definition, especially when you sprint regularly.

There is nothing quite like running in soft sand at BUD/S to challenge your desire to "never quit." It definitely helps to run on the beach prior to reporting to BUD/S because you'll need time to learn the techniques and adjust to the leg fatigue associated with soft-sand running.

To pass these runs, all you have to do is **stay with the pack**. Do not fall behind or you will be further tested through the formation of the GOON SQUAD. The GOON SQUAD is the group that does not stay with the pack on the platoon runs. If by the end of a run a student is not back in formation, they will receive extra physical training in order to "motivate" them. A weekly four-mile timed run on the beach wearing combat boots is a test that will challenge even the best runners. Here are some training tips that will help you decrease your run times and stay with the pack.

RUNNING ON SOFT SAND AND PAVEMENT

When running in the soft sand at BUD/S, stepping in footprints or previously made depressions is the biggest key to success. In soft-sand running, it is essential to change your stride to more of a shuffle and dig your toes into the sand. This will work your calves more than normal pavement running.

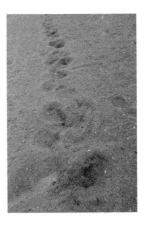

On pavement or hard packed sand, you should find a style of running that feels comfortable and allows you to open your stride efficiently. Decrease the stress on your feet, shins, and knees by landing slightly on the ball of your foot and rolling across your foot through to your toes. You should not be flat footed throughout. This foot strike should land under your body's center of gravity and not out in front of your body. Lean slightly forward to allow for even greater running efficiency.

A good way to check your stride is the audible test. If you can hear your feet hit the ground, you are probably running flat-footed and need to open your stride. Shin splints and stress fractures soon accompany this unnatural style of running. So—run quietly!

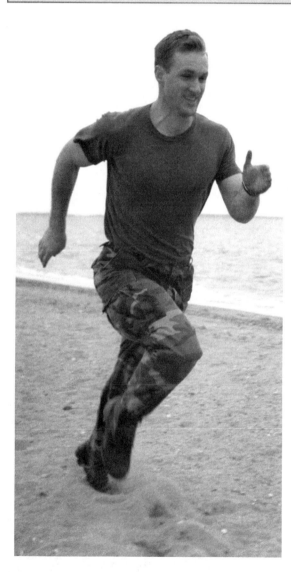

Regardless of the running surface, by far the most important technique of proper running is **breathing**. The proper breath is a very deep inhalation and exhalation. It should feel like a yawn. People who tend to take rapid, shallow breaths create carbon-dioxide build-up, increase their heart rate, and will encourage muscle cramps. Deep breaths get more oxygen to your muscles, rid your body of carbon dioxide, and aid in reducing fatigue.

Relaxing the upper body is another important running technique. When you are running, the only body parts that should be working are your lungs and your legs. If your upper body, fists, or face are clenched or flexed while running, the blood that should be going to your legs is sent to the flexed body parts as well, thus decreasing the amount of oxygen to your legs. Try to relax and breathe deeply.

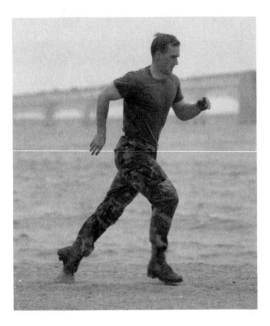

A full arm swing will help you get into a good running step and breathing rhythm. Your hands should swing in a straight line from your hips to your chest. Elbows should be bent slightly and hands should be loose and unclenched.

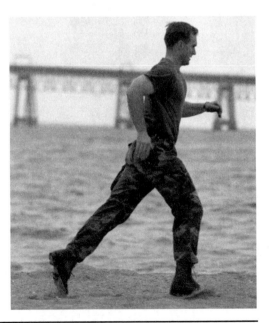

LEARN HOW TO RUN FASTER

Building a foundation of 15–20 miles a week of running is considered to be enough of a foundation to start pushing the envelope on your speed and endurance. If you're not up to this mileage, check out the six-week running plan to build your foundation.

SIX WEEK RUNNING PLAN FOR BEGINNING RUNNERS

	Day 1	Day 2	Day 3	Day 4	Day 5
Week 1	1 to 2 miles	Bike or swim 30 minutes	1 to 2 miles	Bike or swim	1 to 2 miles
Week 2	2 to 3 miles	Bike or swim 30 minutes	2 to 3 miles	Bike or swim	2 to 3 miles
Week 3* no running	Bike or swim 30 minutes	Bike or swim 30 minutes	Bike or swim 30 minutes	Bike or swim 30 minutes	Bike or swim 30 minutes
Week 4	3 miles	Bike or swim 30 minutes	3 miles	Bike or swim 30 minutes	3 miles
Week 5	2 miles	3 miles	Off	4 miles	2 miles
Week 6	2 to 3 miles	3–4 miles	Off	4 to 5 miles	3 miles

* Do not run during Week 3—bike or swim every day instead. There is a high risk of injury to beginners.

INTERVAL TRAINING

Interval training will help you increase your foot speed, build your VO2 Max (which is the maximum amount of oxygen your body can consume during challenging full-body exercises)and will allow you to run at faster paces during your PST distance run—getting you into better shape.

Intervals list your goal time, broken down by ⅛ of a mile sections, to allow you to better pace yourself while running your PST. The chart below is a good reference when you need to find out exactly how fast you need to run.

Running

Interval and Pacing Goal Mile Time Chart

Intervals	Goal mile pace 8:00 mile	Goal mile pace 7:00 mile	Goal mile pace 6:00 mile
½ mile intervals	4:00	3:30	3:00
¼ mile intervals	2:00	1:45	1:30
⅛ mile intervals	1:00	52 seconds	45 seconds

After you have determined how fast you need to run to learn your goal pace, try to run 1 or 2 intervals at a faster than goal pace just to push your limit. After each interval run, walk or slow jog for a recovery for 1 to 2 minutes.

It is most important to learn your pace. You should be able to recognize your breathing, arm swing, leg stride, and foot strikes to create a muscle memory of how you should feel when you are running at your goal pace. As you get into better shape, you should feel better throughout the running event. One day a week, you should push the speed limit and do a series of faster than pace runs.

SUPPLEMENTAL RUNNING PLAN

Feel free to add some runs to **The Complete Guide to Navy SEAL Fitness**'s program if you have a solid running foundation (that is, track, cross-country, or other athletic background).

Unless you are a cross-country runner or track star in high school or college, you will probably have a problem with running a timed run at an above average pace. The reasons for this can range from being a little heavier and stronger in the upper body to simply never having to run under a time limit. (For this, consider long distance running anything in the 1 mile range.)

Anyone can be a faster runner. It takes time, hard speed work, flexibility, and in some cases weight loss. This book is designed to assist with increasing your speed, endurance, and flexibility. This program can be added as a supplement to your current workout program or can replace the running in your program altogether. Naturally, this choice is yours. I would only recommended adding this program to your present program if you have been previously running at least 15–20 miles a week.

When running daily or several times a week, you must follow all stretches thoroughly and perform each for 15 seconds each. This should take you only

RUNNING WORKOUTS

Here are four daily workouts that you can select to increase your running speed. Select one of the following workouts to serve as a supplemental workout, one day a week.

Workout #1:
Run 1 mile at an easy pace.
Stretch.
Repeat 8 to 10 times.
Run ¼ mile at 10 to 20 seconds under current mile pace.
Jog slowly or walk for 1 minute.

Workout #2
Run 1 mile at an easy pace.
Stretch.
Repeat 5 times.
Run ½ miles at 10 seconds under current mile pace.
Jog slowly or walk for 2 minutes.

Workout #3
Run 1 mile at an easy pace.
Stretch.
Run 1 mile at 10 seconds above current mile pace.
Jog for 2 minutes slowly.
Run 1 mile at current mile pace.
Jog for 2 minutes slowly.
Run 1 mile at 10 seconds faster than current mile pace.
Cool down by jogging for 5 minutes.
Stretch.

Workout #4
Run for 5 minutes as a warm-up.
Stretch.
Run for 30 minutes total at the following pace:
1 minute sprint, 1 minute slow jog, repeat.

five minutes, but it's crucial not to miss stretching after a warm-up jog and after your running workout.

Running faster is not a tough goal to achieve if you are presently running a ten minute mile and have an 8 minute mile pace. However, as you can imagine, it's tough to get from a 8 minute mile pace to 6 minute mile pace or faster. It is possible, however, to achieve a 10 minute or 8 minute mile in less than a few months of training if you are not new to running.

For more experienced but slower runners, going from 10 to an 8 minute mile pace is best done with the following recommendations:

8 Week Supplemental Program

Weeks	Monday	Tuesday	Wednesday	Thursday	Friday	Saturday
1 to 4	2 mile run	¼ mile at goal pace. Repeat 6 to 8 times	Rest or PT. Do not run.	1.5 mile timed run and 1.5 mile jog	PACE DAY 3 miles of intervals at goal pace	4 to 6 miles at an easy pace
5 to 8	2 mile run	½ mile at goal pace. Repeat 4 to 5 times	Rest or PT, swim, or bike. Do not run.	2 mile timed run and 2 mile jog	PACE DAY 4 miles of intervals at goal pace	4 to 6 miles at an easy pace

On Mondays, run for two miles. Try to keep at your goal pace for as long as you can. Chart your progress each week to see how far you were able to maintain goal pace.

On Tuesdays, the intervals will help you build your VO2 max and foot speed to better teach yourself your goal pace. On one or two of the interval runs, try to run faster than your goal pace—just to push your limit. After each interval run, walk or jog slowly for recovery for 1 to 2 minutes. During weeks 4 to eight, your distance will increase but your pace will remain the same. Shoot for ½ mile intervals at goal pace.

Wednesday is your day off. Swim or rest. Do your PT exercises today as well as every other day as recommended in this workout program.

On Thursday, test yourself with a timed run. This should be a 1.5 mile timed run and a 1.5 mile jog. Alternatively, try a 4-mile timed run once a month to prep for your BUD/S weekly 4-mile timed run.

On Fridays, you'll learn your pace. All your runs, no matter what the distance, are to be done at your goal pace. Work up to the three mile run. Once you fall off of your pace, stop, walk, and recover for two minutes. Then continue running for shorter intervals until you reach your total distance of three miles.

On Saturday, you'll perform a long run at an easy pace. Have a nice leisurely run at slow moderate pace and stretch well after each running session.

As you can see, the best way to get better or faster at running is to practice running. This routine is aggressive but doable and should only take 20 to 40 minutes on most weekdays.

PREVENT RUNNING INJURIES

Always start off slowly and limit your mileage. If you take off for more than 2 to 3 months from a regular running routine, if you start again "where you left off" you will actually overtrain. You would be running too far, too soon. It takes time to build up to a rigorous amount of running (such as 4 to 6 miles day, 4 to 5 times a week), even if you used to run this far last year.

As I am not a doctor, I like for people to search out information themselves to be better informed. I suggest taking a look at www.drpribut.com, the site of Dr. Steven Pribut. He is a doctor who enjoys running and has a site designed to help describe, prevent, and self-treat the most common running injuries. If your injury does not seem simple and easy to diagnose, go to see your doctor. Here is a short list of the types of injures common to new runners:

- **Shin Splints**—muscular pain in your shins
- **Heel Injuries**—known as Plantar Fasciitis, this is tendonitis in your heel or heel spur
- **ITB Syndrome**—tendonitis on the outside of your knee
- **Runner's Knee**—known as PFS, this is tendonitis on the tendons that connect the kneecap to your leg
- **Achilles Tendonitis**—calf to heel tendon injury that is very painful and serious

All of these pains typically start off as a little twinge while running, then advance to become very painful even when walking. The first thing to do when you experience any of these pains is to stop running, and rest the legs a few days by absolutely no running. You can still cross-train with biking, rowing, swimming, or elliptical gliding. Ice for 10 minutes where it is painful, stop for 1 minute, and repeat the cycle for an hour whenever you can. Taking over-the-counter anti-inflammatory medication is usually okay, but consult a doctor first.

Tips to Prevent Running Injuries

If you are an avid runner, chances are you have experienced at least one injury. In fact, according to Runner's World, over 50% of all runners get injured every year.

In the spring after a winter layoff, or if you are going to start running for the first time, I would recommend the following step up program:

- Stretch for a week prior to actually running to loosen up stiff joints and connective tissue.

- Choose a non-impact aerobic activity like biking, elliptical gliding, rowing, or swimming when you feel the beginnings of an injury. It is never a bad idea to cross-train in any of these activities every other day in place of running.

- Warm-up properly and then stretch. Run nice and easy for about 5 to 10 minutes then stretch again once you are warm and the muscles and joints are more pliable. Never stretch "cold."

- Replace your running shoes often. I go through shoes about every 2 to 3 months and only run in my running shoes. Do not walk in your running shoes since you walk differently than you run. You do get what you pay for. There are a number of types of shoes out there that range from $80–$120. You can save $20–30 by finding them online.

I hope these suggestions can help you prevent some of the common injuries. However, it is always recommended to see a doctor if you are in pain. Two of the running rules I use are: "If it hurts to run—stop running" and "If it hurts to walk—go to a doctor."

SWIMMING AT BUD/S

The sidestroke, or combat swimmer stroke, is the trademark of the U.S. Navy SEALs. This stroke is used for stealth and efficiency. BUD/S students learn the basic stroke in a pool, without fins, and then advance to more challenging environments such as the bay or ocean. The sidestroke is one of the easiest and most effective strokes you will learn. With the sidestroke, you have the advantage of being able to swim as far as six miles and still have the energy to conduct a mission.

SIDESTROKE WITHOUT FINS

Swimming sidestroke without fins requires timing and coordination of kicks, arm pulls, and breathing. Preparing for the SEAL PST 500-yard swim test will be easier if you follow the techniques and recommendations below:

1. **Kick off the wall.** Every length of the pool, turn around, inhale, and kick off the wall, gliding until momentum almost stops. Start exhaling. Then, staying underwater, give one big double-arm pull and glide with your hands by your waist. Angle yourself toward the surface as you glide, because by this time you will need to breathe. When you break the surface to breathe, you should be about 8–10 yards off the wall—with only minimal physical effort!

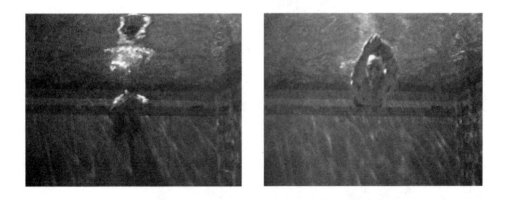

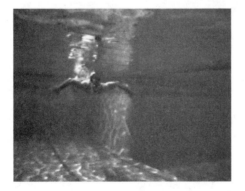

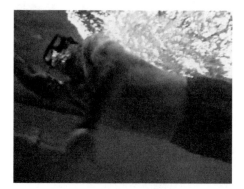
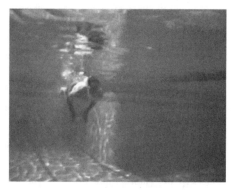

2. **First breath.** Turn to your side and extend your bottom arm over your head. Your top arm remains by your side as you pause for a big inhalation.

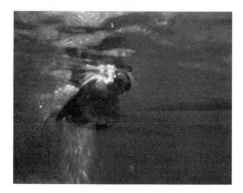
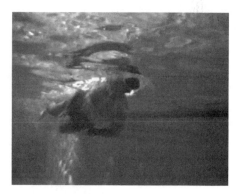

3. **Pull and kick coordination.** As your bottom arm begins its stroke and pulls toward your side (your top arm is already by your side), breathe, then move your arms over your head together. As your arms move forward, your top leg should also move forward as your legs spread to prepare for the big scissor kick.

As you pull your top arm back to your side, kick and exhale at the same time. As your legs come together, the top arm should have completed its stroke and be by your side again as the bottom arm stays extended over your head. This is the glide position. Glide and breathe as you begin to pull your bottom arm to your side again.

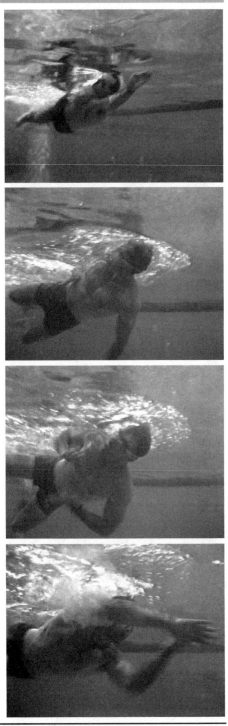

4. **Flutter kick in between scissor kicks are not necessary but will increase speed.** It will also make you more tired, so if you are looking at maxing all of the PST's events, you may want to conserve some energy in the pool and skip the flutter kicks.

SCISSOR KICK

FLUTTER KICK

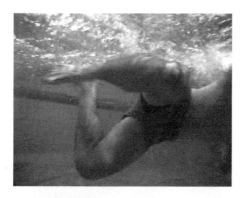

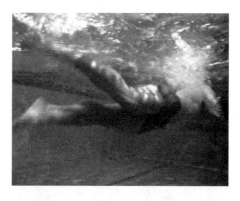

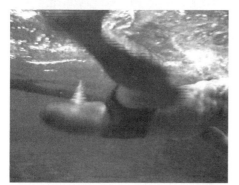

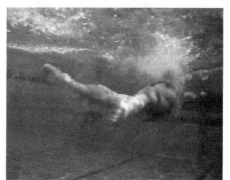

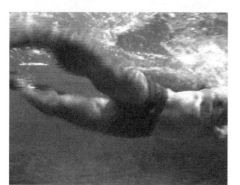

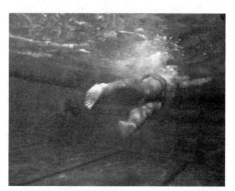

SIDESTROKE WITH FINS

You will use fins 99% of the time once you have entered the First Phase of BUD/S. Your ankles and hip flexors must be strong in order to do this; therefore, I recommend that you are able to swim at least one mile (with fins), without stopping, in less than 30 minutes before arriving at BUD/S. Sidestroke with fins is similar to the sidestroke without fins with only the following differences:

1. **Constant flutter kicks.** With fins on your feet, your biggest source of power will naturally be your legs, so kick constantly in order to be propelled through the water. 90% of your propulsion will come from your legs.

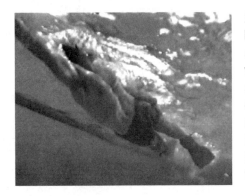

2. **Swimming in a straight line.** About every five to ten strokes, it is important to look forward in order to check if you are swimming in a straight line. This does not need to be done in the swimming pool; however, it is important in the open ocean to have a visual reference when surface swimming to check accuracy.

3. **Arm pull and breathing coordination.** As your top arm completes its stroke and the bottom arm is beginning to pull, breathe. When swimming with fins, your arms play an important role in getting your head above the surface to breathe, but can also be valuable in adding some power to your stroke.

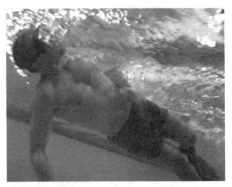

4. **Recovery.** As your bottom arm completes its stroke and is moving forward above your head, your top arm should be moving over your head just ahead of your bottom arm. Keep your top arm close to your body in order to reduce drag.

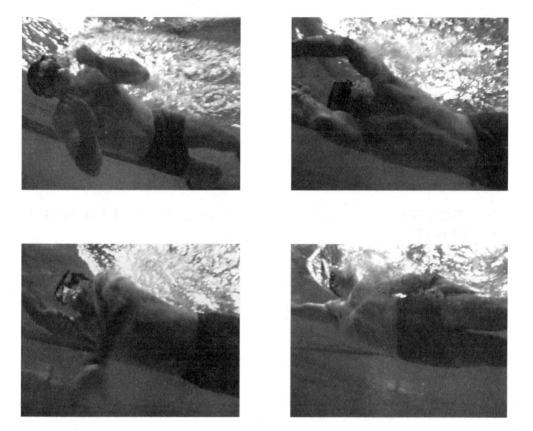

5. **Stretch before you swim.** It is extremely important to stretch your calves, ankles, and feet muscles/tendons before putting on your fins. You will lessen the amount of pain and fatigue in your feet and ankles if you stretch about 10–15 minutes before swimming over a mile in fins.

CRAWLSTROKE (FREESTYLE)

Hypoxic swim training. You will not use the crawlstroke much at BUD/S, but it is a great way to exercise and build your cardiovascular system, especially with hypoxic swimming workouts. The word hypoxic means low oxygen. Adapting this type of workout to swimming is easy, yet will probably be the most challenging cardiovascular exercise you will ever do. Hypoxic swimming easily compares to high-altitude training. Basically, your body is performing with less oxygen because of controlled breath holds while you surface swim. Instead of breathing every stroke or every other stroke, you will hold your breath for up to 10–12 strokes at a time. This gets your body used to performing with less oxygen, resulting in increased endurance when you swim regularly and breathe every stroke.

WARNING: Potentially dangerous—Do not perform alone!

SWIM DRILLS FOR BUD/S EOD (EXPLOSIVE ORDINANCE DISPOSAL), DIVER STUDENTS

These drills are for you to practice prior to getting to advanced diving training.

Tread water. Using your arms and legs, relax and tread water. Try this without using your hands by lifting your hands out of the pool for 5 minutes. Use egg-beater kick for best results At BUD/S you will do this drill with fins and SCUBA gear during dive phase. This requires strong legs used to wearing fins while swimming.

Bottom bounce. With your hands behind you and feet together, bounce off the bottom of the pool 20 times.

Float. Keep your hands and feet in same position and bend 90-degrees at the waist. Float for 10–20 breaths.

Swim. Swim 50–100 yards with your feet and hands in the same position as above. Use the dolphin kick.

Front and back ward flips. Perform flips in the water with hands and feet as in the "Swim" drill above.

Pick up goggles. Dive to the bottom of the pool and picking up goggles or a face mask with your teeth.

Here are a few freestyle tips to help you increase your endurance and break up the monotony of sidestroke swimming.

1. **Kicking off the wall.** In pool swimming, kicking off the wall is essential to building up momentum and reducing the number of strokes per length. With your legs in a full squatting position against the wall, explode in the direction you are swimming and begin 6-inch flutter kicks. Keep your arms extended over your head. As your momentum decreases, begin the single arm pull, and surface to breathe. By this time you should be about 8–10 yards away from the wall.

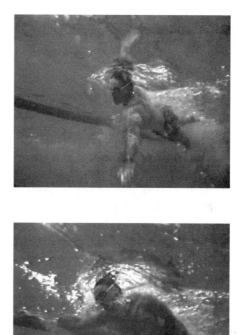

2. **6-Inch Flutter kicks.** Using 6-inch flutter kicks will help you maintain a streamlined position in the water by keeping your body position horizontal. Constant flutter kicks are not necessary, but are recommended for short distance and endurance swimming like you will be doing in this workout.

3. **Arm pulls.** An efficient arm pull is the most powerful and important part of swimming freestyle. The stroke begins with one arm extended over your head and ends when that arm is next to your hip. Each arm opposes the other and is never in the same position or moving in the same direction. As one arm is pulling through the stroke, the other is recovering forward.

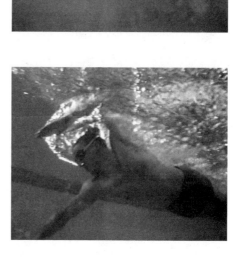

The arm pull is broken down into two parts: the pull and the push. As you pull one arm over your head, bend your elbow slightly and pull your arm under your body about 4–6 inches away from your chest. Once your hand is just below chest level, your pull stroke changes into a push stroke using the triceps muscles in your arm. From your chest, simply straighten out your arm until it brushes past your hips.

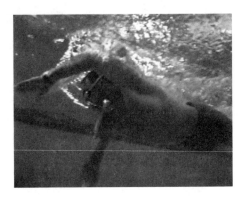

4. **Recovery:** Torso twist and high elbow. After a full arm stroke, recover the arm in front of you by getting your elbow high out of the water. This is aided by slightly twisting your torso in order to get your shoulder and arm out of the water. Breathing requires you to twist your torso at the end of your stroke. Your hand should be by your hip with your other hand extended over your head. This enables you to slightly turn your neck to breathe while still, and most importantly keeping your head in the water. Half of your face should still be underwater when you breathe. This is the most difficult part of freestyle to master—breathing and not lifting your head out of the water.

5. **Keep your head down.** Your body will act like a see-saw in the water. If your head comes out of the water, your lower body will sink, creating more drag and making your stroke much less efficient. A good rule of thumb is to make the water hit the hair line on your head as you glide through the water.

ROPE CLIMBING: JUST FOR FUN

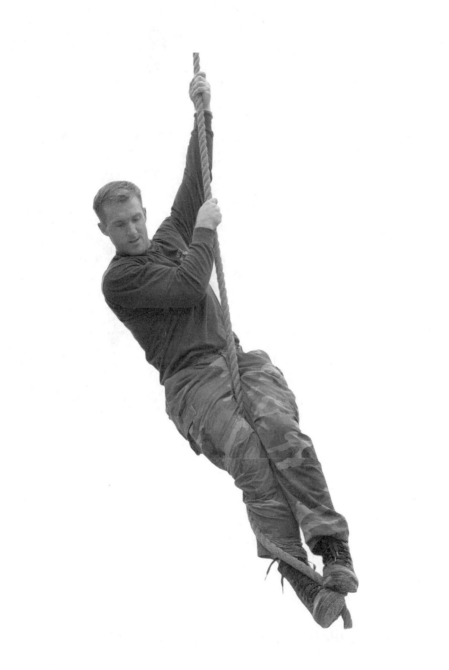

Rope Climbing

BASIC ROPE CLIMBING TECHNIQUES

Using your feet

Wrap the rope around your leg as follows: The top goes at the inner thigh, between your legs, around your knee and calf on the outside of your leg, and across the top of your boot. With the unwrapped leg, clamp your foot on to the rope on the opposite foot. This will act as a brake and you can actually support yourself without using your hands and arms.

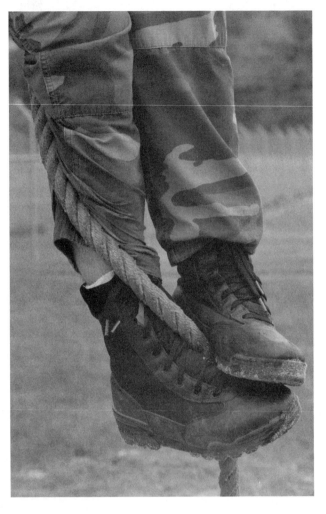

The technique to use so that you do not completely burn out your arms and grip is called the **Brake and Squat Technique.** Climb up the rope by bending your legs, sliding the rope across your foot by loosening the brake foot. Once you have moved about 1–1.5 feet of rope across your foot, brake and straighten your legs. Now you are using your legs to get you up the rope. This does require some amount of upper body strength but will save your energy for the most important part of rope climbing— GETTING DOWN!

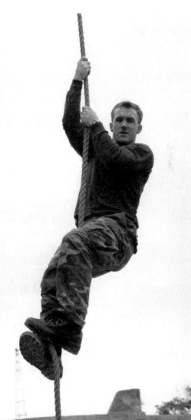

Rope Climbing

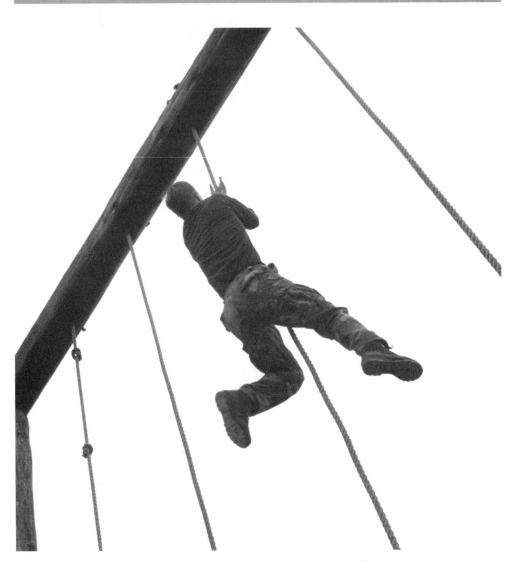

Advanced rope climbing—without your feet on the rope

This method of climbing a rope is a great workout and is absolutely exhausting. Your forearm muscles, biceps and back muscles will scream after a few times of climbing 30 feet of rope without using your legs.

Using a hand over hand method, slowly pull yourself up the rope about 6–12 inches at a time. This method requires an excellent grip (which you can first build by doing pullups) and biceps with stamina.

THE **WORKOUTS**

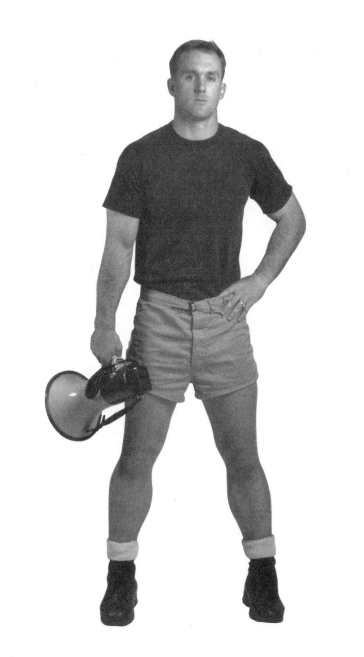

The Complete Guide to Navy Seal Fitness: Third Edition includes three workouts for every level of fitness:

- The 30-Day Beginner's Workout Plan will help any fitness novice quickly lose pounds, preparing them and introducing them to the rigorous activity required by SEAL training.

- The Intermediate Workout is for those accustomed to fitness or sports that need a refresher before leaping into BUD/S training.

- The 12 Weeks to BUD/S workout is a tough workout that will prepare you physically and mentally for the Navy's Basic Underwater Demolition/SEAL training.

This section will explain the types of workouts you'll be performing. Use the following pages as a reference as you go forward on your path to fitness.

THE PT PYRAMID

This workout is deceivingly difficult. The PT Pyramid is unique from any other workout because it has a warm-up, maximum, and a cool down period built into it. Begin climbing the Pyramid on the left side of the base. The levels of the Pyramid are the number of repetitions required in each set. Some exercises will have a (x2) or a (x3) next to the name of the exercise. The repetition number on the pyramid is multiplied by this number, making the workout much more challenging. Usually three or four different exercises are involved in this type of workout.

For example, the first sets of this workout go in this order:

SET #1

Pullups (x1) = 1 rep

Pushups (x2) = 2 reps

Crunches (x3) = 3 reps

SET #2

Pullups (x1) = 2 reps

Pushups (x2) = 4 reps

Crunches (x3) = 6 reps

And onto . . .

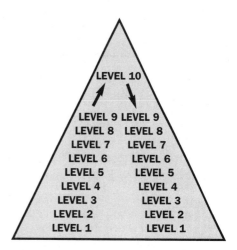

SET #10

Pullups (x1) = 10 reps

Pushups (x2) = 20 reps

Crunches (x3) = 30 reps

Once you reach the top of the pyramid, repeat the numbers and work your way down the right side until you are at the base of the pyramid again. Once you reach the bottom right side of the pyramid, you are finished. If you are beginning a workout program for the first time, do not go on to the following week's workouts until you can successfully complete the entire 19 sets of the pyramid workout.

THREE-MILE TRACK WORKOUT

The track workout is a great way to build speed and endurance for the 1.5-mile run as well as the 4-mile-timed run you will experience weekly at BUD/S. You will begin this interval training program by warming up with a steady one-mile run. This mile should be at a comfortable pace, usually a 7- to 8-minute mile. Run the next 1/4 mile at a full sprint; then jog another 1/4 mile at the same pace you ran the first mile. Repeat the 1/4-mile sprint and 1/4-jog again. Now repeat the same sprint/jog sequence with 1/8 miles four times, totaling another mile of interval training.

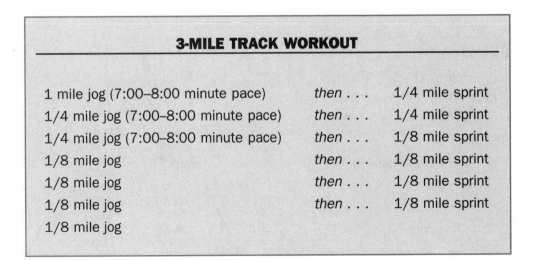

3-MILE TRACK WORKOUT

1 mile jog (7:00–8:00 minute pace)	*then . . .*	1/4 mile sprint
1/4 mile jog (7:00–8:00 minute pace)	*then . . .*	1/4 mile sprint
1/4 mile jog (7:00–8:00 minute pace)	*then . . .*	1/8 mile sprint
1/8 mile jog	*then . . .*	1/8 mile sprint
1/8 mile jog	*then . . .*	1/8 mile sprint
1/8 mile jog	*then . . .*	1/8 mile sprint
1/8 mile jog		

This is not a walking workout. The object of interval training is to catch your breath from running while still moving at a jogging pace. This will speed your recovery time when you are resting. Quicker recovery time means you have more stamina and endurance, and will feel better after rigorous exercise than ever before.

If you have to build yourself up to the above workout by either decreasing the distance or speed, or walking during the jogging portion of the workout, that is fine! The object of this workout is to push yourself, but you can build a foundation by working your way up to the specified times and distances of the 3-Mile Track Workout.

RUN / SWIM / RUN

The Run / Swim / Run workout is one of the best ways to build the endurance you will need for SEAL training. This lower body, cardiovascular exercise program will enable you to build the stamina and endurance needed for increasing your Navy SEAL PST scores. The object of this workout is to run the specified distance as fast as you can and quickly start swimming with little transition time. After swimming, immediately begin running again, and try to match your pace from the first run of the workout.

SWIM-PT

The Swim-PT workout is a quick way to receive a great cardiovascular workout and build muscle stamina at the same time. The challenge of the Swim-PT workout is to swim 100 meters, jump out of the pool, and immediately begin performing pushups and abdominal exercises. After the pushups and situps are completed, jump back in the water and swim 100 meters. Repeat the above sequence for the specified number of sets.

The Workouts

PROPER FULL-BODY WARM-UP

One of the best warm-up routines I do is the jumping jacks/pushups super-set. To really get the heart pumping and the arms warmed up do the following:

- 10 Jumping jacks
- 10 Pushups

Repeat this three to five times. It only takes 2 or 3 minutes each. After warming up, stretch the triceps and chest and shoulders lightly. Make sure to stay on your toes while performing the pushup until you can do pushups no longer. Once you burn out, it is okay to go to your knees in order to finish.

PULLUP WORKOUT

Here's how it works:

	Regular	Reverse	Close	Wide	Mountain Climber Grip
Set #	1–5	6–10	11–15	16–20	21–25
Reps	2,4,6,8,10	2,4,6,8,10	2,4,6,8,10	2,4,6,8,10	2,4,6,8,10
Total	30 reps +	30 reps +	30 reps +	30 reps +	30 reps = 150 reps

The above workout is the most advanced pullup workout of **The Complete Guide to Navy SEAL Fitness**, totaling 25 sets and 150 repetitions of pullups. Before you proceed to the next type of pullups, complete the 5 sets of 2, 4, 6, 8, 10 repetitions of the same type.

SUPER SETS

Most people have never done over 500 pushups and 500 situps in a 30–40 minute workout. Each set of six exercises should be completed within a two-minute period; therefore, the 20 super set workout should be finished within 40 minutes. For example, the 20 super set workout in week #3 is done the following way:

Set #1: 10 Situps → 10 Pushups → 10 Atomic Situps → 10 Triceps Pushups → 10 Leg Levers → 10 Dive Bomber or Wide Grip Pushups Repeat sequence 19 times.

The total number of pushups and abdominal exercises in this workout is 600 (each!). This workout is sometimes referred to as the "Time-Saver" workout. If you are running short on time, you can finish 300 pushups and situps in just 20 minutes. If you are a beginner, I recommend you cut the number of super-sets in half. You will still get 300 repetitions in your workout, but it is important to build a solid base for several months before you attempt to challenge yourself with 600 repetitions of any exercise.

LOWER BODY PT

If you are not used to exercising your legs, you must stretch before, during, and after Lower Body PT. These exercises are explosive and plyometric exercises designed to build speed, strength and endurance. In this workout, you will concentrate on exercises such as frog hops, jumpovers, and lunges, designed to build power in your legs. Whether you are running in boots on soft sand or swimming with fins in the ocean, you will need to have fit and strong legs. If you are not interested in SEAL training, Lower Body PT will build definition in your legs. Perform each exercise the specified number of repetitions, take 15 seconds to stretch, and repeat until all the exercises are complete.

PUSHUP / SITUP / DIP PYRAMID

The object of the Pushup / Situp / Dip Pyramid is to rapidly increase the repetitions in your workout. You will need to perform high repetitions at BUD/S and this is a great way to prepare for hundreds of pushups and situps. The workout goes like this: Begin with pushups and do 20 repetitions the first set. Then, alternate exercises and do 40 repetitions of situps. Next, quickly change to the dip position and perform 15 repetitions. Basically, you are climbing three pyramids at the same time, alternating exercises until you have reached the bottom right of all three pyramids. The toughest set is 50 pushups, 100 situps, and 30 dips.

The Workouts

MINIMAL RUNNING WEEK

Statistically, lower extremity injuries occur during the third week of any running program. Overuse (too much running) or improper preparation will definitely result in injuries to your shins, feet, knees, and/or hips. You should take advantage of this week and stretch well, rest, and ice your joints and shins. You will not get out of shape because you are not running. This week will be challenging because of the amount of swimming you will do to replace the cardiovascular running workout. If you are 100% healthy and an advanced athlete, you may ride a bike for up to one hour in addition to the swimming. It is recommended that you give your legs a break this week, because you will not get a rest in the upcoming weeks.

THE 30-DAY
BEGINNER'S WORKOUT

THE 30-DAY BEGINNER'S WORKOUT PLAN

The 30-Day Beginner's Workout will slowly prepare your body for rigorous activity. It is for true beginners who really need to lose weight more than anything before they start running, lifting, and exercising too rigorously. I would recommend this program for at least 1 to 2 weeks if you were previously in shape, but let yourself slide for 6 to 12 months.

However, if you have not been active ever, or for over five years, or need to lose 30 or more pounds, this 30-Day plan should be followed for an additional 30 says before taking on the challenge of the Navy SEAL Intermediate program.

The 30-Day Beginner's Workout

DAY 1	DAY 2	DAY 3	DAY 4	DAY 5
15:00 walk, run, or bike	**5 sets of:**	20:00 walk, run, or bike	**5 sets of:**	15:00 walk, run, or bike
	10 pushups		10 bicep curls	
	10 crunches		10 triceps extensions	
Full body stretch		Full body stretch		Full body stretch
	Shoulder workout		**Shoulder workout**	
	15:00 walk, run, or bike		15:00 walk, run, or bike	

DAY 6	DAY 7	DAY 8	DAY 9	DAY 10
5 sets of: 3:00 walk, run, or bike 20 squats Full body stretch	15:00 walk, run, or bike **Shoulder workout** Full body stretch	**5 sets of:** 10 jumping jacks 10 pushups Full body stretch	**3 sets of:** 20 squats 10 lunges (each leg) Full body stretch 30:00 walk or bike	15:00 walk, run, bike **Shoulder workout** Full body stretch

The 30-Day Beginner's Workout

DAY 11	DAY 12	DAY 13	DAY 14	DAY 15
15:00 walk, run, or bike	**5 sets of:**	15:00 walk, run, or bike	**5 sets of:**	15:00 walk, run, or bike
75 crunches	10 jumping jacks 10 pushups	75 crunches	10 jumping jacks 10 pushups	75 crunches
Full body stretch	20:00 walk, run, or bike	Full body stretch	20:00 walk, run, or bike	Full body stretch

DAY 16	DAY 17	DAY 18	DAY 19	DAY 20
5 sets of:	15:00 walk, run, or bike	**5 sets of:**	15:00 walk, run, or bike	**5 sets of:**
10 bicep curls 10 triceps extensions 20 squats 10 lunges (each leg)	100 crunches	10 to 20 pushups 20 squats	100 crunches	10 pushups 20 squats 20 crunches
Full body stretch	Full body stretch	Full body stretch	Full body stretch	Full body stretch

The 30-Day Beginner's Workout

DAY 21	DAY 22	DAY 23	DAY 24	DAY 25
20:00 walk, run, or bike	**8 sets of:**	20:00 walk, run, or bike	**5 sets of:**	20:00 walk, run, bike
Shoulder workout	10 jumping jacks 10 pushups	100 crunches	10–15 pushups 20 squats 20 crunches	100 crunches
Full body stretch	30:00 walk, run, or bike	Full body stretch	30:00 walk, run, or bike	Full body stretch
	Full body stretch		Full body stretch	

The 30-Day Beginner's Workout

DAY 26	DAY 27	DAY 28	DAY 29	DAY 30
5 sets of:	**5 sets of:**	20:00 walk, run, or bike	**8 sets of:**	20:00 walk, run, bike
5:00 walk, run, or bike 20 squats 10 lunges (each leg)	10 bicep curls 10 triceps extensions 30 crunches	150 crunches	10 jumping jacks 10 pushups	200 crunches
Full body stretch	Full body stretch	Full body stretch	Full body stretch	Full body stretch

THE INTERMEDIATE WORKOUT

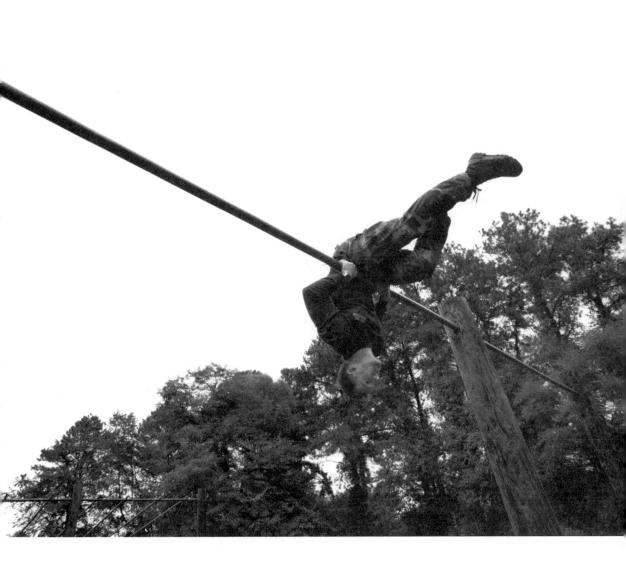

The Intermediate Workout

This workout is not specifically designed for people who are out of shape. However, you can alter some of the workouts to build a foundation in order to move on to the more challenging 12-week workout. First, you can test your level of fitness by taking the SEAL PST.

500 yard swim—If you score above 13 minutes or do not complete:

1. Check your technique by reading Chapter 6 on swimming.

2. Build cardiovascular strength by running, biking, or hypoxic swimming (see Week #2 of the 12-week workout, Thursday).

1.5 mile run—If you score above 13 minutes or do not complete:

1. Check your technique by reading Chapter 5 on running.

2. Do the 3-mile Track Workout (see Week #2 of the 12-week workout, Thursday), except change the words "sprint/jog" to "run/walk."

Pullups—If you do less than 3 pullups:

1. Do negatives to build upper body strength. A negative is half of a complete repetition. Simply put your chin above the pullup bar by stepping up to the bar. Then, slowly let yourself down to the starting position counting to 5. By fighting gravity on the downward motion of the pullup, you are getting your muscles used to lifting your body weight. Eventually, you will be able to lift yourself over the bar.

Pushups—If you do less than 30 pushups in 2 minutes:

1. Do negatives until you can do a full pushup.

2. Do pushups on your knees.

Situps—If you do less than 30 situps in 2 minutes:

1. Do crunches, especially if you have lower back problems.

If you still cannot pass the minimum physical standards on the Navy SEAL PST, you will need to start with the four-week Pre-Training Workout. This is a four-week program that will help you build a foundation of strength and endurance. The workouts may be repetitious, but the best way to build the muscular stamina needed to pass the Navy SEAL PST is by following these simple steps and finishing the four-week program.

Some general guidelines:

1. Work out five days a week and stretch two times every day.
2. Push yourself until you can no longer perform any of the exercises, and then resort to negative repetitions. Pushing yourself to total muscle failure will quickly increase your scores in pull-ups, pushups, and situps.
3. When running or swimming during the Pre-Training phase, concentrate more on perfecting your technique than on decreasing your times.
4. Stretch for 15 minutes after every workout in order to decrease your pain and soreness the following day.

Follow this workout program and you will be surprised that doing 300 pushups and over 500 crunches in one workout isn't as tough as you thought. After your four-week training program is complete, take the SEAL PST again and strive to surpass the minimum scores (see page 21).

GOOD LUCK!

Week #1

MONDAY

Upper Body PT

Regular Pushups 2 x max
  (Do negatives if you
  have to, but stay off
  your knees!)
Wide Pushups 2 x max
Triceps Pushups 2 x max
Regular Pullups
  Do a pyramid to your
  max (for example, if
  your max is 5, do
  1,2,3,4,5)
Reverse Pullups
  Pyramid down to 1
  from your max
Regular Crunches 2 x 25
Reverse Crunches 2 x 25
Left and Right Crunches
  2 x 50 each side

Max pushups in 1 min.
Max situps in 1 min.
Max pullups (no time
  limit)

TUESDAY

Lower Body PT

Squats	2 x 10
Lunges (each leg)	2 x 10
Heel Raises	2 x 10
(each leg)	
Frog Hops	1 x 5

Sprints

20 yd x 5
40 yd x 5
60 yd x 3

Jog 1 mile.
Stretch legs for 15 min.

WEDNESDAY

Running

Jog 1/4 mile.
Stretch 10 min.
1.5-mile timed run.
Jog 1/4 mile.
Stretch 15 min.

THURSDAY

Swimming

Stretch 10 min.
500 yd. sidestroke or
  breaststroke, timed
500 yd sidestroke
  technique swim;
  concentrate on
  technique!
Read Chapter 6 on
  swimming.

FRIDAY

Run/Swim PT

Jog 1/4 mile
Stretch 10 min.
1.5-mile timed run

100 yd swim (freestyle)
10 pushups
10 situps
Repeat sequence 10
times!

SATURDAY

REST!

MONDAY

Upper Body PT

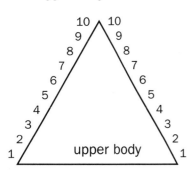

Pullups x 1
Pushups x 2
Situps x 3
Dips x 2
Each level of the pyramid

Running

Jog 1/4 mile
Stretch for 10 min.
2-mile timed run
Jog 1/4 mile
Stretch for 10 min.

TUESDAY

Lower Body PT

Squats	2 x 15
Lunges (each leg)	2 x 15
Heel Raises (each leg)	2 x 15
Frog Hops	1 x 8

Sprints

20 yd x 5
40 yd x 4
60 yd x 3
100 yd x 2

Swimming

500 yds sidestroke
Stretch 10 min.

WEDNESDAY

Running

Jog 1/4 mile
Stretch 10 min.
2-mile timed run
Jog 1/4 mile
Stretch 10 min.

THURSDAY	**FRIDAY**	**SATURDAY**

THURSDAY

Same workout as Monday of this week, but swim 500 yds instead of running—give your legs a break!

After you swim:
Max pushups in 1 min.
Max situps in 1 min.
Max pullups (no time limit)

FRIDAY

Running
Jog 1/4 mile
Stretch 10 min.
2-mile timed run
Jog 1/4 mile
Stretch 10 min.

SATURDAY

REST!

Week #3

Upper Body PT

Pullups:
   1,2,3,4,5...max, and
   then back down to 1
   (15 sec. break in
   between pullups)

10 Super Sets

Regular Pushups	5
Regular Crunches	10
Wide Pushups	5
Reverse Crunches	10
Triceps Pushups	5
1/2 Situps	10

Repeat this sequence 10
times, for a total of
150 pushups and 300
abdominal exercises.
You have 2 min. to
complete each set. If
you finish in 1 min. 30
sec., you have 30 sec.
rest before the next set.

Running

Jog 1/4 mile
Stretch 10 min.
2-mile timed run
Jog 1/4 mile
Stretch 10 min.

Running

3-mile timed run

Swimming

800 yd swim

Lower Body PT

Squats	3 x 15
Lunges	3 x 15
Heel Raises	3 x 15
Frog Hops	2 x 8

Sprints

20 yd x 5
40 yd x 4
60 yd x 3
100 yd x 2
220 yd x 1

THURSDAY

Upper Body PT

Pullups: 1,2,3,4,5...max;
  then back down to 1
  (15 sec. break in
  between pullups)

15 Super Sets

Regular Pushups	5
Regular Crunches	10
Wide Pushups	5
Reverse Crunches	10
Triceps Pushups	5
1/2 Situps	10

Repeat sequence 15
  times,
  for a total of 225
  pushups and 450
  abdominal exercises.

Swimming

500 yd swim

FRIDAY

Running

Jog 1/4 mile
Stretch 10 min.
3-mile timed run
Jog 1/4 mile
Stretch 10 min.

SATURDAY

REST!

Week #4

MONDAY

Upper Body PT

Pullups: 1,2,3,4,5 . . .
  max; then back down to
  1 (15 sec. break in
  between pullups)

15 Super Sets

Regular Pushups	5
Regular Crunches	10
Wide Pushups	5
Reverse Crunches	10
Triceps Pushups	5
1/2 Situps	10

Repeat sequence 15
  times,
  for a total of 225
  pushups and 450
  abdominal exercises.

Running

2–3 miles at a comfortable
  pace

TUESDAY

Running

Jog 1/4 mile
Stretch 10 min.
3-mile timed run

Swimming

1000 yds sidestroke
Stretch 10 min.

WEDNESDAY

Lower Body PT

Squats	3 x 15
Lunges	3 x 15
Heel Raises	3 x 15
Frog Hops	2 x 8

Sprints

20 yd x 5
40 yd x 4
60 yd x 3
100 yd x 2
220 yd x 1

THURSDAY

Upper Body PT

Pullups: 1,2,3,4,5 . . .
max; then back down to
1 (15 sec. break in
between pullups)

20 Super Sets

Regular Pushups	5
Regular Crunches	10
Wide Pushups	5
Reverse Crunches	10
Triceps Pushups	5
1/2 Situps	10

Repeat sequence 200
times,
for a total of 300
pushups and 600
abdominal exercises.

Swimming

500 yds sidestroke

FRIDAY

Running

Jog 1/4 mile
Stretch 10 min.
4-mile timed run
Jog 1/4 mile
Stretch 10 min.

When you have completed the 4-week training program, take the SEAL PST again. You will be surprised at how much your scores will improve. But don't stop there!

After you achieve the minimum scores, I encourage you to keep training, using the 12-week workout. You will soon be in the best physical shape of your life!

THE 12 WEEKS TO BUD/S WORKOUT

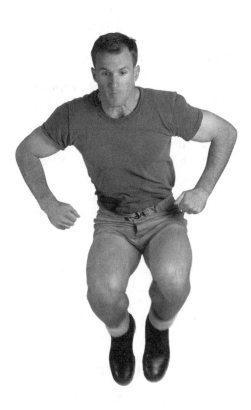

The 12 Weeks To BUD/S Workout

During the 12-week program, you will encounter many types of workouts. Each workout is designed to make you stronger in a different way. I've already briefly explained each workout so you will have a better idea of what to expect during your 12 weeks of intense exercising. In the course of the 12-week program, the structure of the workouts will stay the same, but the difficulty of each workout will grow as the number of repetitions increases. In the 12-week program, I introduce one additional workout.

HYPOXIC SWIM PYRAMID

•*Do not perform this workout alone.*•

The term hypoxic means low oxygen. By holding your breath and surface swimming (freestyle), you will receive a cardiovascular workout like no other. The only comparisons to hypoxic swimming are high-altitude running and cross-country skiing. The reason these workouts are similar is because exercise in high-altitudes, where there is less oxygen in the air, deprives your muscles of the oxygen you need. The same is true for holding your breath while swimming. Lactic acid and fatigue quickly build in your body as you exercise in low oxygen environments; therefore, you can get into much better shape in a shorter amount of time.

After training with a regimented hypoxic swim workout, when you swim normally (breathing every other stroke) your body will have become accustomed to not receiving sufficient oxygen. Thus, you will have more than enough oxygen to feed your muscles, and your performance will be greatly enhanced.

FREQUENTLY ASKED QUESTIONS

How long should I rest in between exercise sets or running and swimming sprints?

Rest as long as you need. Eventually, your rest times should decrease in time and frequency. A good goal is to try to rest about 15–20 seconds between pullup sets. For the swimming sprints and hypoxic workout, try to rest a maximum of 30 seconds before starting again. For running sprints, the rest period will increase as your distance increases if you walk back to the starting line. A 100-yard sprint will give you more rest than a 20-yard sprint.

What strokes should I use during run/swim/run?

I recommend swimming as fast as you can. So try swimming freestyle. If you are training for BUD/S, use the sidestroke (with or without fins).

What counts as a stroke in the hypoxic swim workout?

A stroke in the hypoxic swim workout is one arm movement. When you pull with both arms doing freestyle, that counts as two strokes. The hardest part of this workout is not breathing during the increasing number of strokes.

I'm having trouble in week four. Should I skip to week five?

Yes, if you feel like it. If you are having problems with just one exercise, go on to the next week. If you are having problems with running, swimming, and pullups, you may want to repeat the week causing trouble.

Now you are ready to begin.

Turn the page to face Week #1, and the 12-week challenge...

MONDAY

SEAL PST

500-yd swim: sidestroke
  or breaststroke
pushups: max in 2 min.
situps: max in 2 min.
Pullups: max (no time
  limit)
1.5-mile run: Run in
  combat boots and pants

TUESDAY

Swimming

200m warmup
500m sidestroke
3 x 100m sprints with 20
sec. rest
200m cool down

WEDNESDAY

Running

3-mile timed run
  (sprint 1.5 miles, jog 1.5
miles)

THURSDAY

Swimming

200m warmup
1000m sidestroke
200m cool down

Upper Body PT

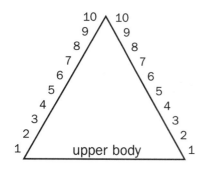

Pullups x 1
Pushups x 2
Situps x 3
each level of the pyramid

Neck exercises

up/down: 20
left/right: 20

8-count Body Builders: 10

Max pushups in 2 min.
Max situps in 2 min.
Max pullups

FRIDAY

Running

4-mile timed run

SATURDAY

Swimming

200m warmup
1000m sidestroke
200m cool down

Week #2

MONDAY

Upper Body PT

Pullups	(sets x reps)
Regular grip	2 x 7
Reverse grip	2 x 7
Close grip	2 x 7
Wide grip	2 x 7
Mountain climbers	2 x 7
Pushups	(sets x reps)
Regular	2 x 15
Triceps	2 x 10
Wide	2 x 15
Dive Bomber	2 x 15
Dips	2 x 15
Arm Haulers	3 x 30

Neck exercises

up/down: 25
left/right: 25

Abdominal PT

Do two cycles of:

Regular situps	40
4-way crunches	40
(Regular, Reverse, Left, and Right: 40 of each)	
Leg levers	40
Flutter kicks	50
1/2 situps	40
Stretch 1 min.	

Running

3-mile timed run (sprint 1.5 miles, jog 1.5 miles)

TUESDAY

Swimming

200m warmup
500m sidestroke
3 x 100m sprints
4 x 50m sprints
200m cool down

WEDNESDAY

Upper Body PT

Pullups	(sets x reps)
Regular grip	2 x 7
Reverse grip	2 x 7
Close grip	2 x 7
Wide grip	2 x 7
Mountain climbers	2 x 7
Pushups	(sets x reps)
Regular	2 x 15
Triceps	2 x 10
Wide	2 x 15
Dive Bomber	2 x 15
Dips	2 x 15
Arm Haulers	3 x 30
8-count Body Builders	15

Neck exercises

up/down: 25
left/right: 25

Abdominal PT

Do two cycles of:

Regular situps	40
4-way crunches	40
(Regular, Reverse, Left, and Right: 40 of each)	
Leg levers	40
Flutter kicks	50
1/2 situps	40
Stretch 1 min.	

Running

4-mile timed run

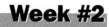

THURSDAY

Swimming

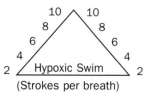

```
        10  /\  10
      8  /    \  8
    6   /      \   6
   4   /        \   4
  2   / Hypoxic  \   2
     /   Swim     \
```

(Strokes per breath)

10 x 50m freestyle with
  10 sec. interval (rest) in
between each 50m
  (Each level of the pyramid is 50m).

DO NOT SWIM ALONE!

Running

3-mile Track Workout
  Jog: 1 mile in 7 min.
  Sprint: 1/4 mile
  Jog: 1/4 mile in 2 min.
  Sprint: 1/4 mile
  Jog: 1/4 mile in 2 min.
  Sprint: 1/8 mile
  Jog: 1/8 mile in 1 min.
  Sprint: 1/8 mile
  Jog: 1/8 mile in 1 min.
  Sprint: 1/8 mile
  Jog: 1/8 mile in 1 min.
  Sprint: 1/8 mile
  Jog: 1/8 mile in 1 min.

FRIDAY

Lower Body PT

Squats	3 x 10
Lunges	3 x 10
Frog Hops	3 x 10
Heel Raises	3 x 15
Jumpovers	3 x 15

Sprints

20m 1/2 pace x 2
20m full sprint x 2
40m 3/4 pace x 2
60m full sprint x 4
100m 1/2 pace x 1
100m full sprint x 2

Neck exercises

  up/down: 25
  left/right: 25

SATURDAY

Swimming

200m warmup
500m sidestroke
3 x 100m sprints (side)
4 x 50m sprints (side)
200m cool down

Running

3-mile timed run

Pullups 5 x 2,4,6,8 reps

  Regular grip
  Reverse grip
  Close grip
  Wide grip
  Mountain climbers
Total Pullups = 100

Abdominal PT

Do two cycles of:
Regular situps	40
4-way crunches	
(40 each way)	40
Leg levers	40
Flutter kicks	50
1/2 situps	40
Stretch 1 min.	

8-count Body Builders 15

Max pushups in 2 min.
Max situps in 2 min.
Max pullups

Week #3

MONDAY

Swim/PT

10 sets of:
100m freestyle
20 pushups
20 abs of choice

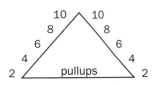

Dips: 25, 20, 15, 10

Neck exercises

up/down: 25
left/right: 25

No running: Due to common overuse injuries such as shin splints and stress fractures, take this week off even if you feel fine.

TUESDAY

Swimming

200m warmup
500m with fins
500m without fins
3 x 100m freestyle sprints at 1 min. 45 sec.
200m cool down

WEDNESDAY

Swim/PT

10 sets of:
100m freestyle
20 pushups
20 abs of choice

Pullups 5 x 2,4,6,8 reps

Regular grip
Reverse grip
Close grip
Wide grip
Mountain climbers

Neck exercises

up/down: 25
left/right: 25

THURSDAY

Swimming

200m warmup
500m with fins
500m without fins
3 x 100m freestyle sprints
   at 1 min. 45 sec.
200m cool down

FRIDAY

Swim/PT

10 sets of:
   100m freestyle
   20 pushups
   20 abs of choice

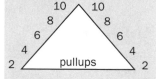

pullups — 10, 8, 6, 4, 2 / 10, 8, 6, 4, 2

Dips: 25,20,15,10

Neck exercises

up/down: 25
left/right: 25

SATURDAY

Running

3-mile timed run
(sprint 1.5 miles,
  jog 1.5 miles)

Swimming

200m warmup
500m with fins
500m without fins

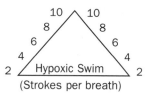

Hypoxic Swim — 10, 8, 6, 4, 2 / 10, 8, 6, 4, 2
(Strokes per breath)

10 x 50m freestyle sprints
at 1 min. 45 sec.
200m cool down

DO NOT SWIM ALONE!

Lower Body PT

Squats	3 x 15
Lunges	3 x 15
Heel Raises	3 x 15
Dirty Dogs	50

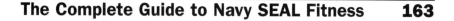
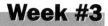

Week #4

MONDAY

SEAL PST

500yd swim: sidestroke
  or breaststroke
pushups: max in 2 min.
situps: max in 2 min.
pullups: max (no time
  limit)
1.5 mile run: Run in
  combat boots and pants

TUESDAY

Run-Swim-Run

Run: 3 miles < 21 min.
Swim: 1 mile with fins
  < 30 min.
Run: 3 miles < 21 min.
Total Time = 1 hr. 15 min.

Neck exercises

up/down: 35
left/right: 35

WEDNESDAY

Upper Body PT

Pullups 5 x 2,4,6,8 reps
  Regular grip
  Reverse grip
  Close grip
  Wide grip
  Mountain climbers
Total Pullups = 100

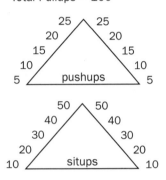

8 count Body Builders: 20

Max pushups in 2 min.
Max situps in 2 min.
Max pullups

THURSDAY

Lower Body PT

Squats	10,15,20
Lunges	10,15,20
Frog Hops	10,15,20
Heel Raises (each leg)	10,15,20
Jumpovers	10,15,20
Dirty Dogs (each leg)	100

Neck exercises

up/down: 35
left/right: 35

Springs

20m 1/2 pace x 2
20m full sprint x 3
40m 3/4 pace x 2
40m full sprint x 3
60m full sprint x 5
80m full sprint x 4
100m full sprint x 3

Swimming

200m warmup
500m sidestroke
500m freestyle
500m with fins
200m cool down

FRIDAY

Running

5 miles < 35 min.

SATURDAY

Upper Body PT

Pullups 5 x 2,4,6,8 reps
  Regular grip
  Reverse grip
  Close grip
  Wide grip
  Mountain climbers
Total Pullups = 100

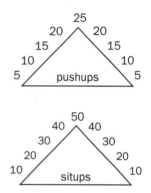

Neck exercises

up/down: 35
left/right: 35

8-count Body Builders: 20
Max pushups in 2 min.
Max situps in 2 min.
Max pullups

Swimming

2000m with fins

Week #5

MONDAY

20 Super Sets:

Triceps Pushups	10
Regular Situps	7
Pushups	10
Reverse Crunches	7
Wide Pushups	10
1/2 Situps	7

Do 20 cycles of all six
exercises. You have 2
min. to perform each
cycle.
Total time: 40 min.
Total Pushups: 600
Total Abs: 420

Upper Body PT

Pullups: 16, 14, 12
Dips: 25, 20, 15
8-count Body Builders:
20, 15, 10

Neck Exercises:

up/down: 40
left/right: 40

Swimming

Swim with fins: 30 min.
Swim continuously for at
least 1 mile

TUESDAY

Run-Swim-Run

3-mile run
1-mile swim without fins
3-mile run

WEDNESDAY

Lower Body PT

Squats	3 x 15
Lunges	3 x 15
Frog Hops	2 x 10
Jumpovers	2 x 20
Heel Raises	3 x 20
Dirty Dogs	3 x 50

Sprints

20m x 5
40m x 5
60m x 5
100m x 4
200m x 2
440m x 1

Swimming

Hypoxic Swim
(Strokes per breath)

11 x 100m freestyle
without fins. 15 sec.
rest in between each
100m.
DO NOT SWIM ALONE!

Neck exercises:

up/down: 40
left/right: 40

THURSDAY

Upper Body PT

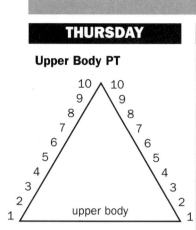

Pullups x 1
Pushups x 2
Abs of choice x 3
Dips x 2
Each level of the pyramid

Flutter kicks 100
Leg Levers 100
8-count Body Builders 25

Neck exercises:

up/down: 40
left/right: 40

Run-Swim-Run

3-mile run
1-mile swim without fins
3-mile run

FRIDAY

Swimming

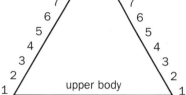

(Strokes per breath)

11 x 100 freestyle without fins. 15 sec. rest in between each 100m.

DO NOT SWIM ALONE!

Running

3-mile Track Workout
Jog 1 mile in 7 min.
Sprint 1/4 mile
Jog 1/4 mile in 2 min.
Sprint 1/4 mile
Jog 1/4 mile in 2 min.
Sprint 1/8 mile
Jog 1/8 mile in 1 min.
Sprint 1/8 mile
Jog 1/8 mile in 1 min.
Sprint 1/8 mile
Jog 1/8 mile in 1 min.
Sprint 1/8 mile
Jog 1/8 mile in 1 min.

SATURDAY

Upper Body PT

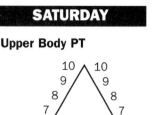

Pullups x 1
Pushups x 2
Abs of choice x 3
Dips x 2
Each level of the pyramid

Flutter kicks 100
Leg Levers 100

Neck exercises:

up/down: 40
left/right: 40

Week #6

MONDAY

10 Super Sets

Pullups	8
Pushups	20
Abs of choice	20
Dips	10

Abs Super Set x 2

Hanging Knee Ups	10
Regular situps	30
Oblique crunch	30
(left and right)	
30 each side	
Atomic situps	30
Crunches	30
Reverse crunches	30

Neck exercises:

up/down: 40
left/right: 40

Swimming

Swim continuously for 45
   min. with fins.
   Goal: 1.5–2 miles

Running

4-mile Track Workout
Jog 1 mile in 7 mins.
3 sets of:
   Sprint 1/4 mile
   Jog 1/4 mile in 1 min.
   45 sec.
6 sets of:
   Sprint 1/8 mile
   Jog 1/8 mile in 1 min.

TUESDAY

Swimming

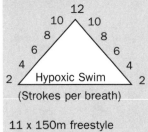

(Strokes per breath)

11 x 150m freestyle
   without fins. 15
   sec. rest in
   between each 200m

DO NOT SWIM ALONE!

WEDNESDAY

Lower Body PT

Squats	4 x 15
Lunges	4 x 15
Frog Hops	3 x 15
Jumpovers	3 x 20
Heel Raises	4 x 20
Dirty Dogs	2 x 100

Sprints

20m x 5
40m x 5
60m x 5
100m x 5
200m x 3
440m x 2

Swimming

Swim continuously for 45
   min. with fins
   Goal: 1.5–2 miles

Running

4-mile Track Workout
Jog 1 mile in 7 min.
3 sets of:
   Sprint 1/4 mile
   Jog 1/4 mile in 1 min.
   45 sec.
6 sets of:
   Sprint 1/8 mile
   Jog 1/8 mile in 1 min.

THURSDAY

10 Super Sets

Pullups	8
Pushups	20
Abs of choice	20
Dips	10

8-count Body Builders: 5
Max pushups in 2 min.
Max situps in 2 min.
Max pullups

Neck exercises:

up/down: 40
left/right: 40

Abs Super Set x 2

Hanging Knee Ups	10
Regular situps	30
Oblique crunch	30
(left and right)	
30 each side	
Atomic situps	30
Crunches	30
Reverse crunches	30

Swimming

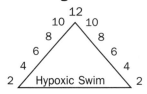

11 x 150m freestyle without fins. 15 sec. rest in between each 200m.

FRIDAY

Swimming

Swim continuously for 45 min. with fins.
Goal: 1.5–2 miles

SATURDAY

Upper Body PT

Pullups: 4 x 2, 4, 6, 8, 10
Regular grip
Reverse grip
Close grip
Wide grip

Pushups: 50,40,30,20,10
Dips: 30,25,20,15,10
8-count Body Builders:
25,20,15,10

Max pushups in 2 min.
Max situps in 2 min.
Max pullups

Neck exercises:

up/down: 40
left/right: 40

Abs Super Set x 2

Flutter kicks 100
Leg Levers 100
Situps 100

Week #7

MONDAY

SEAL PST

500yd swim: sidestroke or
    breaststroke
pushups: max in 2 min.
situps: max in 2 min.
pullups: max (no time
    limit)
1.5 mile run: Run in
    combat boots and pants

TUESDAY

Run-Swim-Run

Run 4 miles
Swim 3000m with fins
Run 3 miles

Lower Body PT

Squats	3 x 15
Lunges	3 x 15
Frog Hops	2 x 10
Jumpovers	2 x 20
Heel Raises	3 x 20
Dirty Dogs	3 x 50

Neck exercises:

up/down: 50
left/right: 50

WEDNESDAY

Swimming

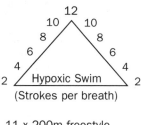

(Strokes per breath)

11 x 200m freestyle
without fins. 15 sec.
rest in between each
200m.

DO NOT SWIM ALONE!

THURSDAY

Upper Body PT

Pullups:

Regular grip	2 x 7
Reverse grip	2 x 7
Close grip	2 x 7
Wide grip	2 x 7
Mountain climbers	2 x 7

Pushups:

Regular	2 x 30
Triceps	2 x 20
Wide	2 x 30
Dive Bomber	2 x 30

Dips	2 x 25
Arm Haulers	3 x 50
8-count	
Body Builders	2 x 20

Max pushups in 2 min.
Max situps in 2 min.
Max pullups

Neck exercises

up/down: 50
left/right: 50

Abs Super Set x 2:

Regular situps	60
4-way crunches	50
Leg levers	60
Flutter kicks	150
1/2 situps	100

Stretch 1 min.

Running

5-mile timed run

Swimming

1 mile swim with fins

FRIDAY

Running

Run 6 miles.

SATURDAY

Run-Swim/PT-Run

Run 4 miles.
15 sets: Swim/PT
   20 pushups
   20 abs of choice
   100m swim
Run 3 miles.

Week #8

MONDAY

Upper Body PT

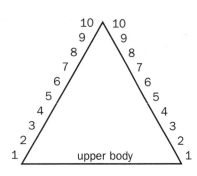

Pullups x 1
Pushups x 3
Abs of choice x 5
Dips x 2

Run-Swim-Run

Run 4 miles.
Swim 1 mile with fins.
Run 3 miles.

Neck exercises:

up/down: 2 x 35
left/right: 2 x 35

TUESDAY

Lower Body PT

Squats	4 x 20
Lunges	4 x 20
Frog Hops	3 x 20
Jumpovers	3 x 20
Heel Raises	4 x 20
Dirty Dogs	2 x 100

Running

4-mile Track Workout
Jog 1 mile in 7 min.
3 sets of:
Sprint 1/4 mile in
1 min. 20 sec.
Jog 1/4 mile in
1 min. 45 sec.
6 sets of:
Sprint 1/8 mile in 40
sec.
Jog 1/8 mile in 1 min.

Swimming

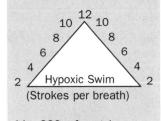

11 x 200m freestyle
without fins. 15 sec.
rest in between each
200m.

DO NOT SWIM ALONE!

WEDNESDAY

Swimming

Swim with fins 1.5 miles.

Neck exercises

up/down: 2 x 35
left/right: 2 x 35

THURSDAY

Run-Swim/PT-Run

Run 3 miles.
10 sets: Swim/PT
  100m sprints
  25 pushups
  25 abs of choice
Run 3 miles.

Max pushups in 2 min.
Max situps in 2 min.
Max pullups

FRIDAY

Upper Body PT

Pullups: 5 x 2,4,6,8,10
  Regular grip
  Reverse grip
  Close grip
  Wide grip
  Mountain climber
Total Pullups: 150

Arm Haulers: 2 x 75

Neck exercises:

up/down: 2 x 35
left/right: 2 x 35

Abs Super Set

Flutter kicks 150
Leg Levers 150
Situps 150

Swimming

Swim with fins 1.5 miles.

Running

Run 4 miles in 27 min.,
in sand if available.

SATURDAY

Running

Run 6 miles within 40 min.

Upper Body PT

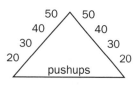

50   50
40   40
30   30
20   20
pushups

100   100
80   80
60   60
40   40
situps

30   30
25   25
20   20
15   15
dips

Week #9

Upper Body PT

Pull-ups: 5 x 2,4,6,8,10
  Regular grip
  Reverse grip
  Close grip
  Wide grip
  Mountain climber

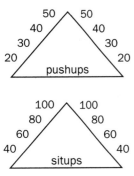

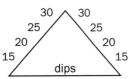

Arm Haulers: 2 x 75

Neck exercises:

  up/down: 2 x 40
  left/right: 2 x 40

Run-Swim-Run

Run 4 miles.
Swim 1 mile with fins.
Run 3 miles.

Lower Body PT

Squats	4 x 20
Lunges	4 x 20
Frog Hops	3 x 20
Jumpovers	3 x 20
Heel Raises	4 x 20
Dirty Dogs	2 x 100

Sprints

20m x 5
40m x 5
60m x 5
100m x 5
200m x 3
440m x 2

Swimming

200m warmup
500m pulls (no kick)
300m kicks (no pull)
8 x 50m sprints
  (15 sec. rest
  between each)
2 x 100m sprints
  (20 sec. rest
  between each)
Hypoxic: 4,6,8,10
  (strokes/breath)
  x 100m
200m cool down

Run-Swim-Run

Run 4 miles.
Swim 1 mile with fins.
Run 4 miles.

Neck exercises

  up/down: 2 x 40
  left/right: 2 x 40

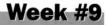

THURSDAY

Swimming

200m warmup
500m pulls (no kick)
300m kicks (no pull)
8 x 50m sprints
  (15 sec. rest between
  each)
2 x 100m sprints
  (20 sec. rest between
  each)
Hypoxic: 4,6,8,10
  (strokes/breath) x 100m
200m cool down

FRIDAY

Lower Body PT

Squats	4 x 20
Lunges	4 x 20
Frog Hops	3 x 20
Jumpovers	3 x 20
Heel Raises	4 x 20
Dirty Dogs	2 x 100

Running

Run 4 miles in 27 min.

Swimming

Swim 2000m with fins.

SATURDAY

Upper Body PT

Pull-ups: 5 x 2,4,6,8,10
  Regular grip
  Reverse grip
  Close grip
  Wide grip
  Mountain climbers

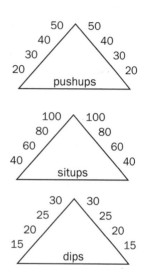

Neck exercises

up/down: 2 x 40
left/right: 2 x 40

Running

3-mile timed run.
(spring 1.5 mile, jog 1.5
  mile)

MONDAY

SEAL PST

500yd swim: sidestroke or breaststroke
pushups: max in 2 min.
situps: max in 2 min.
pullups: max (no time limit)
1.5 mile run: Run in combat boots and pants

TUESDAY

Running

Run 4 miles in 27 min.

WEDNESDAY

Upper Body PT

Pull-ups: 2,4,6,8,10 x 5
    Regular grip
    Reverse grip
    Close grip
    Wide grip

Arm Haulers: 2 x 75

20 Super Sets

Situps	10
Pushups	10
Atomic situps	10
Triceps	10
Leg Levers	10
Dive Bombers	10

Run-Swim-Run

Run 3 miles.
Swim 1 mile with fins.
Run 3 miles.

THURSDAY

Lower Body PT

Squats	3 x 20
Lunges	3 x 20
Frog Hops	3 x 15
Jumpovers	3 x 20
Heel Raises	3 x 20
Dirty Dogs	2 x 100

Sprints

20m x 5
40m x 5
60m x 5
100m x 5
200m x 3
440m x 2

FRIDAY

Running

Run 5 miles in 33 min.

SATURDAY

Swim/PT

15 sets of:
Freestyle springs: 100m
Pushups: 15
Abs of choice: 15

Max pushups in 2 min.
Max situps in 2 min.
Max pullups

Arm Haulers: 2 x 75

Swimming

Swim 2 miles with fins.

Week #11

MONDAY	TUESDAY	WEDNESDAY

MONDAY

Upper Body PT

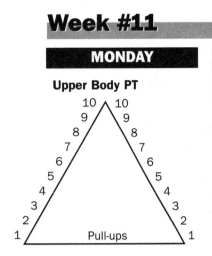

10 / 10
9 / 9
8 / 8
7 / 7
6 / 6
5 / 5
4 / 4
3 / 3
2 / 2
1 / 1
Pull-ups

25 Super Sets

Situps	10
Pushups	10
Atomic situps	10
Triceps	10
Leg Levers	10
Dive Bombers	10

Neck exercises:

up/down: 2 x 50
left/right: 2 x 50

Swimming

1-mile swim with fins

TUESDAY

Running

4-mile timed run

WEDNESDAY

Swim/PT

Hypoxic swim
5 x 50 at 50 sec. intervals
   (6 strokes/breath)
4 x 50 at 55 sec. intervals
   (8 strokes/breath)
3 x 50 at 1 min. intervals
   (10 strokes/breath)
2 x 50 at 1 min. intervals
   (12 strokes/breath)
1 x 50 (no breaths)

DO NOT DO ALONE!

Swim PT

10 Sets of:
   100m sprint (freestyle)
   15 pushups
   15 abs of choice

Neck exercises:

up/down: 2 x 50
left/right: 2 x 50

THURSDAY

Running

4-mile timed run

FRIDAY

Swimming

1-mile swim with fins

Upper Body PT

Pull-ups: 5 x 2,4,6,8,10
   Regular grip
   Reverse grip
   Close grip
   Wide grip

Arm Haulers: 2 x 75

Neck exercises:

   up/down: 2 x 50
   left/right: 2 x 50

20 Super Sets

Situps	10
Pushups	10
Atomic situps	10
Triceps	10
Leg Levers	10
Dive Bombers	10

SATURDAY

Running

3-mile timed run
   (sprint 1.5 mile, jog 1.5
   mile)

Week #12

20 Super Sets

Triceps Pushups	10
Regular Situps	7
Regular Pushups	10
Reverse Crunches	7
Wide Pushups	10
1/2 Situps	7

Total Time: 40 min.
Total Pushups: 600
Total Abs: 420

Pull-ups: 16, 14, 12
Dips: 25, 20, 15

Running

4-mile timed run

Swimming

Hypoxic swim
  5 x 50m,
   50 sec. intervals
  4 x 50m,
   55 sec. intervals
  3 x 50m,
   1 min. intervals
  2 x 50m,
   1 min. intervals
  1 x 50m

DO NOT SWIM ALONE!

The number of breaths per 50m = number of times you swim the 50m; i.e., 5 x 50m means you swim 50 meters five times on only 5 breaths...

Running

4-mile timed run

THURSDAY

Swim/PT

10 sets of:
  100m freestyle sprint
  20 pushups
  20 abs of choice

Upper Body PT

Pull-ups: 5 x 2,4,6,8,10
  Regular grip
  Reverse grip
  Close grip
  Wide grip

Arm Haulers: 2 x 75

FRIDAY

Running

3-mile timed run

SATURDAY

Swimming

Hypoxic swim
  5 x 50m,
  50 sec. interval
  4 x 50m,
  55 sec. interval
  3 x 50m,
  1 min. interval
  2 x 50m,
  1 min. interval
  1 x 50m

DO NOT SWIM ALONE!

STEW'S TOP TEN LIST

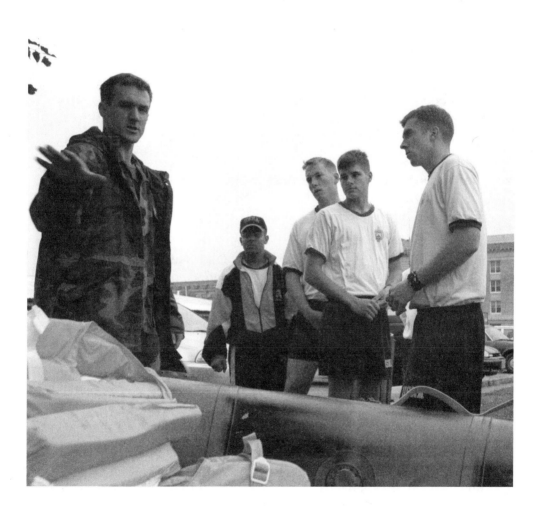

The Top Ten Before BUD/S

HERE ARE THE TOP TEN THINGS YOU NEED TO DO BEFORE YOU GO TO BUD/S

1. **Arrive fit!** Not just able to do the minimum scores but Stew Smith's recommend PST scores:

500 yds swim	under 9:00
Pushups	100 in 2:00
Situps	100 in 2:00
Pullups	20
1.5 mile run	under 9:00

    If you need letters of recommendation from SEALs, most SEALs will not endorse you unless you can achieve the above numbers. Do this book two to three times and I guarantee you will be able to hit these scores. Sometimes it takes a solid year of training.

2. **Run in boots and swim with fins!** At least 3–4 months prior to arriving at BUD/S, get the legs used to swimming with fins and running in boots. They issue Bates 924s and UDT or Rocket Fins at BUD/S.

3. **Officers at BUD/S:** Go there ready to lead and get to know your men. Start the team-building necessary to complete BUD/s. You can't do everything by yourself, so learn to delegate but do not be too good to scrub the floors either. Be motivated and push the guys to succeed. Always lead from the front.

4. **Enlisted at BUD/S:** Be motivated and ready to work as a team. Follow orders but provide constant feedback so your team can be better at overcoming obstacles that you will face. Never be late!

5. **BUD/S is six months long!** Prepare for the long term, not the short term. Too many people lose focus early in their training and quit. It would be similar to training for a 10K race and running a marathon by accident. You have to be mentally focused on running the marathon—in this case a six month "marathon."

6. **Weekly physical tests:** The four mile timed runs are weekly and occur on the beach—hard packed sand next to the water line. They are tough, but not bad if you prepare properly.

   The 2 mile ocean swims are not bad either if you are used to swimming with fins when you arrive. The obstacle course will get you to if you are not used to climbing ropes and doing pullups. Upper body strength is tested to the max with this test.

7. **Eating at BUD/S:** You get three great meals a day at BUD/S, usually more than you can eat. During Hellweek, you get four meals a day—every six hours! The trick to making it through Hellweek is just make it to the next meal. Break up the week into several six hour blocks of time.

8. **Flutterkicks:** This seems to be a tough exercise for many. Practice 4 count flutterkicks with your ab workouts and shoot for sets of at least 100. There maybe a day you have to do 1000 flutterkicks. By the way—that takes 45 minutes!

9. **Wet and Sandy:** Jumping into the ocean then rolling around in the sand is a standard form of punishment for the class at BUD/S. It is cold and not comfortable, so you just have to prepare yourself for getting wet and sandy everyday at BUD/S. On days that you do not get wet and sandy, it will be the same feeling as getting off early at work on a three day weekend!

10. **Did I mention running?** You should be able to run at least 4 miles in 28 minutes in boots with ease. If not you will so learn to hate the "goon-squad." The goon squad is to motivate you never to be last again or fail a run.

Any more questions—you can reach me at Stew@stewsmith.com or the www.getfitnow.com website message boards.

HOW TO BECOME
A NAVY SEAL

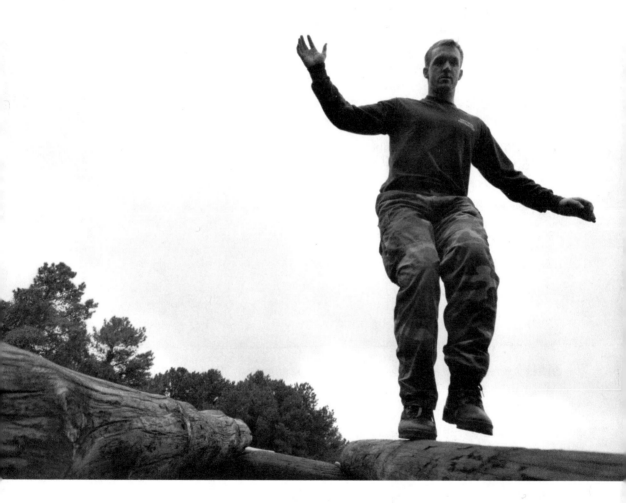

How to Become a Navy SEAL

Becoming a SEAL is challenging. In some cases, it may actually be harder to enter SEAL training than to graduate from SEAL training. This is primarily in the officer ranks, though. Unfortunately, the Navy SEALs do not need officers as much as enlisted personnel, so naturally it will be tougher to become an SEAL officer. The most unusual aspect of SEAL training is that the officers and enlisted participate in the same training. This is very rare in the Navy. In fact it is rare in the entire military. Perhaps this is one reason for the closeness of the SEAL units. It creates an environment of mutual respect.

Before you can enter the SEAL program you must meet the following general requirements:

EYESIGHT: Your eyesight may be no worse than 20/40 in one eye and 20/70 in the other, and it must be correctable to 20/20 with no color blindness. You may have a waiver if vision is 20/70 in one eye and 20/100 in the other, correctable to 20/20. A waiver is also needed for people who get PRK surgery prior to enlisting.

ACADEMIC TESTS: The required ASVAB score is: VE + AR = 104, MC = 50. You may be eligible for a waiver (up to 5 points). Handled on a case-by-case basis.

PHYSICAL TESTS: The BUD/s Physical Screening Test (PST)

500 yd sidestroke / breaststroke swim (10:00 rest)

Max pushups in 2:00   (2:00 rest)

Max situps in 2:00   (2:00 rest)

Max pullups   (10:00 rest)

1.5 mile run in boots and pants

AGE: Applications are accepted from men who are 28 years old or less. You may request an age waiver (for those 29–30); however, the age waivers are reviewed on a case-by-case basis.

U.S. CITIZEN: The program is only open to men, and you must be a U.S. citizen for security-clearance requirements.

You can enter into the SEAL program right out of high school at the age of 18 or you can go to college or work and still enlist into the SEAL program up to the age of 28. There are age waivers, but they are few and far between and are handled on a case-by-case basis by the Commanding Officer of BUD/S and the SEAL Community Manager.

Many college graduates enlist instead of entering as an officer mainly due to the large number of officer candidates who apply and the small number who get accepted. The Navy needs more enlisted men than officers in the SEAL Teams basically. Last numbers were one out of every eight who apply get accepted in the officer program.

Another reason why it is challenging to become an officer right out of college is due to the number of college graduates in the enlisted ranks who also place requests for Officer Candidate School. The Navy has a choice of selecting a SEAL veteran enlisted with a college degree or a 22 year old college kid with little experience. That is why many select to enlist right out of college instead of becoming an officer immediately. If you want to be a SEAL, this is a great way to get experience. AND you do not have to go through BUD/s again!

You can enlist either the conventional way or via the SEAL Contract. When you enlist in the U.S. Navy under the SEAL contract, you must sign a contract that states you are giving a certain number of years in return for a guaranteed job. When you enlist under the SEAL Challenge contract, you are guaranteed orders to BUD/S as long as you are qualified and pass a PT screen test in Boot Camp. Everyone who volunteers to take the BUD/S screening test is allowed to take the test at Bootcamp—SEAL Challenge enlisted or the conventional enlisted.

There are advantages to signing the SEAL Challenge Contract. By signing, you are enlisting with the intent of becoming a SEAL. This means that you don't have to worry about getting orders to BUD/S as long as you pass the PT screen test in Boot Camp. This also means that you get four chances to pass the PT screen test at Great Lakes.

If you enlist under any other contract, you are not guaranteed a billet at BUD/S and may have to go to the fleet and complete a minimum tour of duty (which is two years) before requesting an inservice transfer to Naval Special Warfare—BUD/S. You can volunteer at Boot Camp and you may get orders to BUD/S, but it's not guaranteed.

NEW CHANGES TO SEAL RECRUITING AS OF OCTOBER 2006

If you think you have what is takes to become a member of Naval Special Warfare or Special Operations, you now have several choices. In October

2006, the Navy changed the way SEAL Teams, SEAL recruits, and all the branches of Naval Special Warfare/Operations do business. Now, SEAL enlisted personnel no longer have to select Source ratings (i.e. BM, RM, GM etc) and learn a job that they will not practice as SEAL operators. The Special Warfare and Special Operations communities have their own rating source codes and the training is considered their A school. If you're looking to be a member of Naval Special Warfare/Operations community, you have four choices:

1. Naval Special Warfare/SEAL (Sea, Air, Land)
2. Naval Special Warfare/SWCC (Special Warfare Combatant Crewman)
3. Naval Special Operations/EOD (Explosives Ordinance Disposal)
4. Naval Special Operations/Diver (Deep Sea Diving and Salvage Operations)

This change in structure not only affects the way SEALs operate but also how Navy Divers, EOD, and SWCC operate as well. Now, if a member gets injured at SEAL Training or decides the SEALs are not for him, he can transfer into one of the other special warfare or special operations professions. If the student has the desire and meets the standards of the other communities in SpecWar/SpecOps, he can attend one of those schools. All the SpecWar/Spec Ops communities are seeking to expand their size by up to 20% by 2010. A student will also be able to choose another career path within the Navy. Here are the four steps required to becoming a member of the Navy Special Warfare/Operations community:

Step 1: Choose a Spec Ops/Spec War Source Rating

Competition for rank advancement occurs within the Special Warfare community as opposed to competing Navy-wide for advancement to the next pay grade. All Naval Special Warfare/Naval Special Operations careers have individual source ratings. A recruit will attend boot camp with one of the following designations, and as long as he can pass the Physical Screening Test at boot camp, he can attend the next phase of training.

SEAL (Sea, Air, Land): (SO)

SWCC (Special Warfare Combatant Crewman): (SB)

EOD (Explosive Ordinance Disposal): (EOD)

Diver: (ND)

Step 2: Training (using SEAL candidate training only as an example)

No longer do boot camp graduates have to go to a variety of A schools. Now, all of the above members of the Special Warfare/Operations Communities use their own training as their A school. For instance, a SEAL recruit will go straight to BUD/S—Basic Underwater Demolition/SEAL training after boot camp and a SWCC recruit will go to SWCC training to learn their job and rating.

Here is the SEAL recruit training pipeline:

- BUD/S Indoctrination: (5 weeks, Coronado, CA)
- BUD/S Phase I: Physical conditioning (2 months, Coronado, CA)
- BUD/S Phase II: Diving (2 months, Coronado, CA)
- BUD/S Phase III: Weapons, demolitions and small unit tactics (2 months, Coronado, CA)
- Parachute Jump School: (1 month, Ft. Benning, GA)
- Advanced Sea, Air and Land Training: (5 months, Coronado, CA)

Step 3: Advanced Training/Placement (SEAL Community)

Upon graduation, the new SEAL will receive their Naval Special Warfare Classification and further opportunities for Advanced Training. The new recruit will report to a SEAL Team or SEAL Delivery Vehicle (SDV) Team in Virginia Beach, VA, Pearl Harbor, HI or Coronado, CA. For up to the first six months, the new SEAL will have an opportunity to continue Individual Specialty Training or they can choose to join a SEAL platoon/SDV Task Unit and continue work-up training to prepare for future deployments.

Step 4: Deployment and Combat Operations

After an intense workup with your SEAL/SDV Platoons, you will be deployable for international operations. Typically, SEALs will deploy with their team to an area of operations around the world and then conduct a variety of small unit missions.

HOW TO PREPARE FOR NAVAL SPECIAL WARFARE/OPERATIONS TRAINING

Due to the Naval Special Warfare mission of increasing the size of the Naval Special Warfare/Operations up to 20% by 2010, the Navy has hired former Navy SEAL, Divers, and EOD members to help recruiters in every recruiting district screen, recruit, and prepare young recruits both mentally and physically for the various SpecWar/SpecOps schools. Ask your local recruiter about the Navy Special Warfare/Special Operations Mentor in your area. The mentor's duties are to help you prepare for training by giving regularly scheduled Physical Screening Tests (PSTs) and other workouts that consist of:

- 500 yard swim (using sidestroke, breaststroke, or combat swimmer stroke)
- 2 minutes of Pushups (max reps)
- 2 minutes of Sit-ups (max reps)
- 2 minutes of Pullups (max reps)
- 1.5 mile timed run (wearing PT gear/running shoes and SEALs wearing boots/cammies)

There are basic minimum scoring standards for this Physical entrance exam, but keep in mind that if you are planning just for the minimums, you have a six percent chance of graduating. Strive for above averages scores and be in top shape before reporting. This will require months—maybe even a year or two—to get into SpecWar/SpecOps Shape.

NAVAL SPECIAL WARFARE IS LOOKING FOR THE MENTALLY TOUGH

Some say that SEAL training is 10% physical and 90% mental. What does that actually mean? It means you'll be pushed physically past your point of exhaustion, making you dig deep within yourself to let your body perform even when you have nothing left. This is where the 90% mental comes into play. You have to mentally will yourself past this point of exhaustion so you can finish your mission. It truly is a test of mind over matter. As you know "if you don't mind—it doesn't matter."

To properly prepare for BUD/S, you do not need to lift heavy weights in the gym, do martial arts for hours a day, soak your body in freezing water, or sleep in the backyard in the winter. All you need to do to prepare for the rigors of high repetition PT, miles of running, swimming with fins, and obstacles courses is climb rope, run, swim, PT and take your showers or baths in water that is 60–70 degrees Fahrenheit. No need to soak in ice. Water in Southern California ranges about 50–70 degrees year round.

Becoming SCUBA qualified prior to BUDS/ EOD/DIVER is not a bad idea. Using a regulator for the first time during diving phase can be a bit intimidating. You will have to learn dive physics and dive medicine, so an understanding of math and the science of diving will be beneficial to any SPECWAR/SPECOPS recruit. See a PADI or NAUI Scuba School near you, though it is not a necessity.

If you think you have what it takes, see a local recruiter and they will link you up to a SpecWar/SpecOps mentor to prepare you for a very challenging career.

PACKAGE SUBMISSION PROCESS

If you are in the Navy and wish to change jobs and become a SEAL, the requirements for submitting a BUD/S training application package are as follows:

Submit through your chain of command a "Special Request Chit" requesting BUD/S training. Then see your Command Career Counselor to begin the process outlined below.

Submit to SPECWAR/Diver Assignment a "Personnel Action Request" (Form 1306/7). Include the following with your request:

- A certified copy of your ASVAB test scores

- Your physical screening test results

- Pressure and oxygen tolerance test results (if completed)

- Your completed diving physical

- (Form SF88 - SF93)

- Your medical record documenting that all immunizations and HIV results are up to date

- A certified copy of your last performance evaluation report

- Make a copy of your entire package and keep the copy in a safe place.

Mail your package to the address below.

SPECWAR/Diver Assignment
BUPERS PERS401D1
5720 Integrity Drive
Millington, TN 38055-0000
Phone: (901) 874-3622
DSN: 882-3622

You may be an officer or enlisted in another branch of service. There are a few inter-service transfers a year and they are handled on a case by case basis. Many times you have to serve your enlistment with the Marines or Army, get discharged from the service and reapply to the Navy. Most of the time, you do not have to do Bootcamp over again. Your best start on this process is to contact the above number of the SpecWar Detailer in Tennessee.

NEW SPECIAL WARFARE DIVISION IN BOOT CAMP

If you are thinking about joining the SEAL or SWCC communities, the Navy has a great offer for you. Sign up under the SEAL Challenge and specify you want to ship to Great Lakes on a certain date. When you get to boot camp, you will be enrolled in a Special Warfare division with other recruits desiring placement in the Navy's special warfare/special operations communities.

What are the benefits?

You will get the opportunity to PT in preparation for the SEAL/SWCC screen test. (Note: You should be able to pass before going to Bootcamp, which will ensure you don't get out of shape.)

You will wear a special T-shirt denoting your status as a member of the Special Warfare Division.

You will be mentored by members of the Dive Motivator's office to make sure your career is a success.

Special Warfare personnel will give you special briefings on their community.

WHAT DO I HAVE TO DO?

If you are ready to make that all-important decision and enlist, see your local recruiter. If you want to be a SEAL or SWCC, make sure you enlist under the SEAL Challenge. If you aren't ready to enlist by July 2 you can still come into the Navy under the SEAL Challenge contract, which will guarantee that if you can pass the screen test you will go to BUD/S.

RECRUITERS:

Points of Contact

SEAL Recruiter West Coast
Naval Special Warfare
2446 Trident Way
San Diego, CA 92155-5494
Com. (619) 437-2049 / 437-5009
DSN 577-2049 / 5009
FAX: Com. (619) 437-2018
DSN 577-2018 SEAL Recruiter East Coast

NSWC DET Little Creek
1340 Helicopter Rd.

Norfolk, VA 23521-2945
Com. (757) 363-4128
DSN 864-4128
More information at:
www.getfitnow.com message boards
www.sealchallenge.navy.mil
www.stewsmith.com SEAL Detailer

SPECWAR/Diver Assignment
BUPERS PERS401D1
5720 Integrity Drive
Millington, TN 38055-0000
Com. (901) 874-3622
DSN 882-3622 Dive Motivators (SEAL)
BLDG 1405

Recruit Training Command
Great Lakes, IL 60088
Com. (847) 688-4643
DSN 792-4643
Toll-free Info Line: 1-888-USN-SEAL

MASTERING THE SEAL PHYSICAL SCREENING TEST

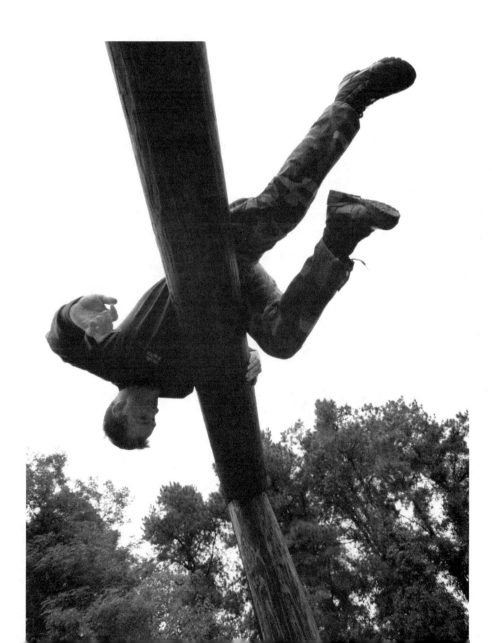

MASTERING THE SEAL PHYSICAL SCREENING TEST!

First of all—the SEAL PST was developed to test swimming and running capability and upperbody muscle stamina—all of which are vital to becoming a Navy SEAL. The following is designed to help you master the test by demonstrating techniques in training as well as test taking. You need a strategy when taking the SEAL PST.

Test yourself. The anxiety felt by young SEAL wanna-be's and other service members is largely due to performing within a time limit. The more your workouts are timed the better you are at "pacing" yourself, thus eliminating most anxiety. By practicing the PST often, you will develop a pace and know when to push yourself at the right times.

THE SWIM:

The 500 yard swim—is what eliminates most people who want to become SEALs. You may pass this part of the test, but you may also completely burn yourself out for the upperbody portion and the run in the process. Here are the test techniques I recommend to score the best time possible while saving your stamina for the pullups, pushups, situps and run:

Kick off the wall and glide as far as you can. You must train using the hypoxic swim pyramid found in this workout to build up your cardiovascular system. You will be winded but you will save yourself several strokes per length.

Strokes per length—the most important factor of the swim. If you can swim a 9:00 swim, that is great. But if it takes you 12–14 strokes per length (25 yards) to do it, you are wasting your energy. On the other hand, if you can swim a 9:00 swim with 6–7 strokes per length you will save over 150 arm strokes and kicks in the process. This is called swimming efficiency! By swimming more efficiently, you will have more energy for the upperbody portion and the run.

How do you get more efficient?

Kick off the wall, double arm pull and glide. Then glide each stroke out after the top arm pull and the kick/recovery to its fullest. Time yourself the old way and then time yourself the new gliding way. You will find that your scores will be the same even though it "feels" like you are swimming slower. You are not swimming slower, you are swimming more efficiently. I recommend an average glide time of 2–3 mississippi's.

PUSHUPS AND PULLUPS—SAME STRATEGY:

Pushups—Placing your hands in the wrong position can seriously affect your maximum score. A perfect location for your hands is just outside shoulder width. This position enables the chest, shoulders and triceps to be equally taxed. Keep hands at shoulder height when in the up position. Your pushups will be weakened if your hands are too low, wide, close or high...in the Navy SEAL pushup test, you are allowed to shake out your arms, as long as one hand and both feet are on the ground. The best way to take this test is to do as many as you can as fast as you can. Then rest in the up position, shake off one arm, repeat with the other arm. Then continue to pump out small sets of 5–10 pushups, shaking it out after every set.

Pullups—During the pullup and pushup test, you want to perform these as fast as possible while adhering to the proper form and technique. The slower you perform these exercises, the more gravity will affect your best score possible. In other words, do not waste your energy returning to the down position. Just let yourself fall. The faster you perform these exercises, the more you will be able to do. Also, look straight up at the sky in order to use your back muscles more for pullups. Pyramid workouts with these exercises will enhance your test scores significantly. The key to training for this part of the test is to keep doing pullups and pushups until you fail. You will succeed in your failure!

SITUPS:

This is an exercise you need to pace. Most people burn out in the first 30 seconds with 30 sit-ups accomplished, only able to perform another 20 or so situps within the next 1:30. By setting a pace at, for instance, 20 situps every 30 seconds, you can turn your score of 50–60 to 80 with very little effort. 25 situps in 30 seconds will give you the score of 100 situps in 2:00.

Mental Games—When I take the test, I always count in my head small numbers like 1–5 or 1–10. I never say eleven or twenty-one. The reason behind this is I feel I am starting over again every time I say "one". This may work for some, it may not. It has helped many in the past.

Mastering the SEAL Physical Screening Test

THE RUN:

For most people the most challenging event of any PST is by far the run. I receive many requests everyday from military members who are seeking workouts for their 1.5 mile, two or three mile PST runs (Navy/ Army/Marine Corps respectively). Since all these distances use relatively the same training philosophy—short distance, faster pace—here are a few options to help all Armed Forces members, regardless of service, get a little faster on their runs.

Timed run—PACE—The most important thing is to not start off too fast. Start off too fast and you will burn out and probably fail the run. Learn your pace and set your goal by pacing yourself to the finish. For instance, if your goal is to run the 2 mile run in 14:00, you must run a 7:00 mile or a 1:45 1/4 mile... For you SEAL wanna-be's, if you want to run a 9:00 1.5 mile test score, you need to start out and finish with a 90 second 1/4 mile. Keep this pace and you will have a 9:00 score.

Recommended workout and techniques—The Four Mile Track Workout has worked for many military and short distance runners for years. This workout is basically interval training. Interval training means you run at a certain pace for a particular distance then increase the pace for the same distance.

The Four Mile Track Workout is broken into 1/4 mile sprints and jogs and 1/8 mile sprints and jogs for a total of four miles. The workout goes as follows:

4 Mile Track Work

>   Jog—1 mile in 7:00–8:00

Three sets of:

>   Sprint-1/4 mile
>   Jog—1/4 mile in 1:45

Six sets of:

>   Sprint-1/8 mile
>   Jog—1/8 mile 1:00

Do this workout without walking to rest. The only rest you will receive is during your slower jogging pace. Try to catch your breath while you jog. Have fun with this one; it is tough.

Another good speed workout is called REPEATS. Simply run a certain distance as fast as you can a specified number of times. This time you get to walk to recover and catch your breath before the next sprint. You can try one of the following distances for a challenging workout:

Mile repeats

1 mile x 3–4 (walk 1/2 mile in between) = 3–4 miles

1/2 mile repeats—

1/2 mile x 6 (walk 1/4 mile in between) = 3 miles

1/4 mile repeats—

1/4 mile repeats x 12 (walk 1/8 mile in between) = 3 miles

1/8 mile repeats—

1/8 mile repeat x 16 (walk 100 yds in between) = 2 miles

Finally, if you have not had enough, you can try mixing shorter jogs and sprints together for a longer period of time. This type of training is great for building the speed and endurance needed for any of the PSTs or 5 or 10K races. I call them SPRINT / JOGS. Simply run about 50 yards as fast as you can then jog 50 yards fairly slow in order to catch your breath. I like doing this one where telephone poles line the road so I can just sprint to one telephone pole then jog to the next.

Sprint / Jogs

50 yd sprint / 50 yd jog for 10, 20, 30 minutes

All of these workouts are fantastic ways to get faster but build the needed endurance which most sprinters lack. Remember to take big deep breaths, relax your upperbody and slightly bend your arms. Do not run flat footed.

These are the techniques to ace the SEAL PST and any other physical fitness test. Many members of the FBI, Marine RECON, Army Special Forces and Navy SEALs have utilized these techniques and went from wanna-be to their dream job. Good luck. If you have any questions, you can reach me on the www.get-fitnow.com web boards or at stew@stewsmith.com.

ABOUT THE AUTHOR

Former Navy SEAL Lieutenant Stew Smith, CSCS, graduated from the United States Naval Academy in 1991 and received orders to Basic Underwater Demolition/SEAL (BUD/S) training. He graduated BUD/S Class 182 as Class Leader and went on to write workouts that prepare future BUD/S students for BUD/S, which are still in use today by SEAL recruiters. His writings include *The BUD/S Warning Order* and the books *The Complete Guide to Navy SEAL Fitness*, *Maximum Fitness*, *The Special Operations Workout*, *The SWAT Workout*, and many other books, guides, and professional fitness programs.

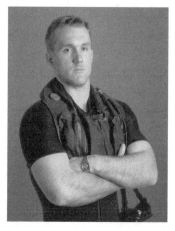

Stew Smith has been featured on many television shows with his fitness products such as National Geographic Channel's *Fight Science*, ABC's *The View* and others. He has been covered in newspaper and magazine articles such as *Sports Illustrated*, *Men's Health*, *Police Mag*, the *Los Angeles Times*, *The New York Times*, *Washington Times*, and many others.

HEROES OF TOMORROW FITNESS

Stew Smith created Heroes of Tomorrow Fitness, a program dedicated to helping future military, law enforcement and fire fighters ace physical fitness tests. Acing your tests requires strategy and daily effort and Stew Smith can show you how to arrive more fit so you can better focus on your job. Email Stew Smith at stew@stewsmith.com if you have any questions about the workout or any other fitness related issue.

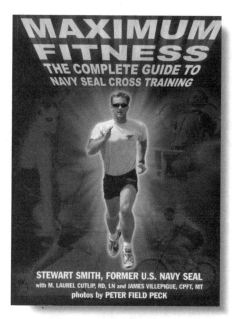

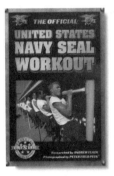
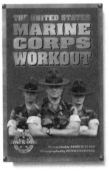
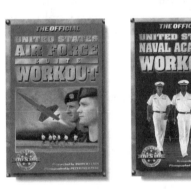

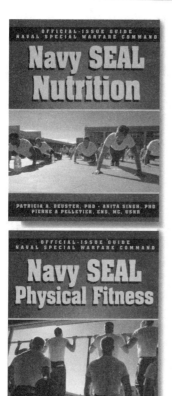